Bilio-Pancreatic Malformations in Adult Patients

Bilio-Pancreatic Malformations in Adult Patients

By

Houssem Harbi, Nozha Toumi
and Nouha Dammak

Cambridge
Scholars
Publishing

Bilio-Pancreatic Malformations in Adult Patients

By Houssem Harbi, Nozha Toumi and Nouha Dammak

This book first published 2023

Cambridge Scholars Publishing

Lady Stephenson Library, Newcastle upon Tyne, NE6 2PA, UK

British Library Cataloguing in Publication Data
A catalogue record for this book is available from the British Library

ISBN (10): 1-5275-2540-6
ISBN (13): 978-1-5275-2540-5

TABLE OF CONTENTS

List of Illustrations xi

List of Tables xiii

Preface xv

List of Abbreviations xvii

Part 1: Cystic Dilation of Bile Ducts

Chapter 1: Introduction 3

Chapter 2: History 5

Chapter 3: Epidemiology 7
1. Frequency 7
2. Sex-Ratio 7
3. Age 7

Chapter 4: Classification of CDBD 9
1. Todani Classification 9
1.1. Type I 9
1.2. Type II 10
1.3. Type III 10
1.4. Type IV 11
1.5. Type V 12
1.6. New Type VI 15
2. Other Classifications 16
2.1. Visser Classification 16
2.2. Modified Todani Classification 18

Chapter 5: Pancreatico-Biliary Maljunction 21
1. Definition of PBMJ 21
2. Classifications of PBMJ 22
2.1. Komi Classification 22

2.2. Kimura Classification 24
2.3. Japanese Classification of 2015 24

Chapter 6: Anatomopathological Study 25
1. Macroscopic Study 25
1.1. Volume of Choledochal Cyst 25
1.2. Choledochal Cyst Wall 25
1.3. Choledochal Cyst Contents 25
2. Microscopic Study 26

Chapter 7: Clinical Presentation 27
1. Circumstances of CDBD Discovery 27
2. Clinical Manifestations 27
2.1. Abdominal Pain 27
2.2. Jaundice 28
2.3. Right Hypochondrium Mass 28
2.4. Other Clinical Signs 29
2.5. Main Complications 29

Chapter 8: Biological Findings 31
1. Blood Count 31
2. Liver Tests 31
3. Pancreatic Enzymes Assay 31

Chapter 9: Imagery 33
1. Abdominal Ultrasound 33
2. Abdominal CT-Scan 34
3. Magnetic Resonance Cholangiopancreatography (MRCP) 35
4. Bilio-Pancreatic Endoscopic Ultrasound 38
5. Endoscopic Retrograde Cholangiopancreatography (ERCP) 39
6. Percutaneous Transhepatic Cholangiography 39
7. Biliary Scintigraphy 40
8. Intraoperative Cholangiography 40

Chapter 10: Evolution and Complications 43
1. Infectious Complications 43
1.1. Acute Cholangitis / Infection of Cyst Contents 43
1.2. Acute Cholecystitis 44
2. Mecanical Complications 44
2.1. Biliary Lithiasis 44
2.2. Rupture of Choledochal Cyst 44

2.3. Compression of Neighbouring Structures 45
2.4. Acute Pancreatitis.. 45
3. Secondary Biliary Cirrhosis.. 46
4. Malignant Degeneration.. 46

Chapter 11: Treatment of CDBD.. 49
1. The Treatement Objectives.. 49
2. Therapeutic Methods 49
2.1. Medical Treatement.. 49
2.1.1. Correction of Metabolic Disorders 49
2.1.2. Antibiotherapy in Case of Bile Infection 49
2.2. Endoscopic Treatment.. 50
2.3. Interventional Radiology.. 50
2.4. Surgical Treatment 50
2.4.1. Surgery Approaches.. 50
2.4.2. Surgical Methods.. 51
2.4.2.1. The Old Methods 51
2.4.2.2. The Reference Methods 52
3. Treatment Indications 53
3.1. Indications for Surgical Treatment...................................... 53
3.1.1. CDBD Type I.. 54
3.1.2. CDBD Type II 54
3.1.3. CDBD Type III... 54
3.1.4. CDBD Type IV... 55
3.1.5. CDBD Todani Type V 55
3.1.6. CDBD (New) Type VI.. 56
3.1.7. PBMJ 56
3.1.8. Enterobiliary Anastomosis after Choledochal Cyst Resection 57
3.2. Indications for Endoscopic Treatment.................................. 60
3.3. Special Cases... 60
3.3.1. In an Infectious Context.. 60
3.3.2. CDBD and CBD Lithiasis... 60
3.3.3. CDBD and Cirrhosis... 61
3.3.4. Cholangiocarcinoma Arising in CDBD 61
3.3.5. CDBD with Gallbladder Agenesis.................................. 61

Chapter 12: Prognosis.. 63
1. Mortality 63
2. Morbidity 63
2.1. Early Complications.. 63

2.2. Late Complications 64

Chapter 13: Conclusion 67

Part 2: Pancreatic Ducts Anomalies

Chapter 1: Introduction 73

Chapter 2: The Pancreas Divisum 75
1. Epidemiology 75
2. Embryology 75
3. Associated Biliopancreatic Anomalies 79
4. Pathogeny of Acute Pancreatitis due to PDIV: 79
5. Symptomatology 81
6. Imaging and Diagnostic Modalities 82
6.1. Abdominal CT Scan 82
6.2. Magnetic Resonance Cholangiopancreatography (MRCP) 83
6.3. Endoscopic Ultrasound (Eus) 86
6.4. Does ERCP Contribute to the Diagnosis Of PDIV? 87
7. Treatment 89
7.1. Aims and Principles 89
7.2. Non Interventional Treatment 89
7.3. Endoscopic Treatment 90
7.4. Surgical Treatment 98
7.4.1. Decompressive Surgical Procedures 99
7.4.1.1. Trans Duodenal Sphincteroplasty 99
7.4.1.2. Puestow Procedure 100
7.4.2. Resection Procedures 101
7.4.2.1. Conventional or Pylorus Preserving Duodenopancreatectomy (CD-PPDP) 102
7.4.2.2. Head Pancreatic Resection with Duodenal Preservation (HPRDP) 102
7.4.2.3. Pancreatic Head Resection with Segmental Duodenal Resection (PHRSD) 103
7.4.2.4. Total Dorsal Pancreatectomy (TDP) 104
7.4.2.5. Total Pancreatectomy with Islet Auto-Transplantation 105
7.5. Endoscopic Versus Surgical Procedures 105

Chapter 3: The Annular Pancreas 107
1. Embryogenesis 107
2. Clinical Presentation 110
3. Imaging 111
3.1. Annular Pancreas in Neonates and Infants 112
3.2. The Upper GI Series 112
3.3. Duodenoscpy and ERCP 112
3.4. CT-Scan and CPRM 113
3.5. Imaging of the Peri-Portal Annular Pancreas 115
4. Treatment 116
4.1. Treatment of Duodenal Obstruction 116
4.2. Treatment of Acute Pancreatitis 117

Chapter 4: Agenesis of the Dorsal Pancreas 119
1. Embryogenesis 119
2. Epidemiology 119
3. Clinical Presentation 120
4. Imagery 120
5. Treatment 122

Chapter 5: Ansa Pancreatica 123
1. Epidemiology 124
2. Clinical Signs 126
3. Imaging 127
4. Treatment 128
4.1. Medical Treatment 128
4.2. Endoscopic Sphincterotomy of the Minor Papilla 128

Chapter 6: Conclusion 131

References 135
Part 1: Cystic Dilataion of Bile Ducts 135
Part 2: Pancreatic Ducts Anomalies 147

LIST OF ILLUSTRATIONS

Part 1: Cystic Dilation of Bile Ducts

Figure 4-1: The 3 subgroups of CDBD type I according to the Todani classification 10
Figure 4-2: The type II of CDBD according to the Todani classification 10
Figure 4-3: The type III of CDBD according to the Todani classification 11
Figure 4-4: The type IV of CDBD according to the Todani classification 12
Figure 4-5: Morphological characteristics that Todani's classification is based on 13
Figure 4-6: Todani classification of CDBD 14
Figure 4-7: Visser's classification of CDBD 17
Figure 4-8: Modified Todani classification proposed by Kronfli R et al. 19
Figure 5-1: Komi classification of AJBPs 23
Figure 5-2: Japan's 2015 BPA classification 24
Figure 9-1: Abdominal ultrasound images showing a choledochal cyst 34
Figure 9-2: MRCP showing a PBMJ type Ia of the Komi classification and type A of the Japanese classification 35
Figure 10-1: MRCP showing an area of bile duct thickening 47

Part 2: Pancreatic Ducts Anomalies

Figure 2-1: Pancreas divisum embrypgenesis 76
Figure 2-2: Types of pancreas divisum 78
Figure 2-3: Ct-scan showing pancreas divisum with chronic pancreatitis. 82
Figure 2-4: MRCP showing an incomplete pancreas divisum 84
Figure 2-5: MRCP showing an inverted pancreas divisum 85
Figure 2-6: Two and 3 dimensions images of MRCP showing a complete pancreas divisum with intra ductal stones 86
Figure 2-7: ERCP image showing complete pancreas divisum. 88

Figure 2-8: Endoscopic views showing endoscopic sphincterotomy of the minor papilla. 92
Figure 2-9: Surgical procedures for the management of the pancreas divisum 99
Figure 2-10: Minor papilla trans duodenal sphincteroplasty 100
Figure 2-11: Puestow procedure: Latero-lateral pancreatojejunal anastomosis 101
Figure 2-12: Surgical resection procedures 103
Figure 2-13: Nakao technique 104
Figure 3-1: Theories of annular pancreas formation 108
Figure 3-2: Abdominal CT-scan showing the “crocodile jaw” sign suggesting the dignosis of an annular pancreas. 113
Figure 3-3: MRCP showing an annular pancreas. 115
Figure 4-1: Abdominal CT-scan showing corporeo-caudal agenesis of the pancreas 121
Figure 4-2: MRCP showing corporeal caudal agenesis of the pancreas 121
Figure 5-1: Ansa pancreatica formation 123
Figure 5-2: Ansa pancreatica type 1 124
Figure 5-3: Ansa pancreatica type 2 124
Figure 5-4: MRCP showing an ansa pancreatica 127
Figure 5-5: Rendez-vous technique 129

LIST OF TABLES

Part 1: Cystic Dilation of Bile Ducts

Table 4-1: Percentage of CDBD types (according to the Todani classification) in different North African series 15
Table 9-1: MRI aspects of the most frequent Todani types of CDBD (part 1) 37
Table 9-2: MRI aspects of the most frequent Todani types of CDBD (part 2) 38
Table 9-3: MRCP and intraoperative cholangiography aspects of some types of CDBD 41
Table 11-1: Results of studies comparing HDS and AHJ 59
Table 11-2: Results of studies about HDS 60

Part 2: Pancreatic Ducts Anomalies

Table 2-1: Definitions of response to endoscopic treatment of symptomatic PDiv (part 1) 94
Table 2-2: Definitions of response to endoscopic treatment of symptomatic Pdiv (part 2) 95
Table 2-3: Definitions of response to endoscopic treatment of symptomatic Pdiv (part 3) 96
Table 2-4: Definitions of response to endoscopic treatment of symptomatic Pdiv (part 4) 97
Table 2-5: Outcomes of total dorsal pancreatectomy for pancreas divisum: published case reports 105
Table 3-1: Types of annular pancreas according to Yogi classification 109
Table 5-1: Incidence of ansa pancreatica in the literature 125

PREFACE

Ductal anomalies of the biliary and pancreatic ducts are congenital malformations that can remain asymptomatic for a long time and are thus diagnosed in adulthood particularly in case of complication.

The biliary atresia is the only biliary malformation that appears at birth and will not be dealt with in this manuscript. On the other hand, we will focus in this book only on bilio-pancreatic malformations in adults that are:

- Cystic dilation of the bile ducts
- Bilio-pancreatic maljunction
- Pancreas divisum: the most common pancreatic ductal anomaly
- The annular pancreas
- Dorsal agenesis of the pancreas and
- Ansa pancreatica (the least frequent malformation)

It is worth noting that the advent of MRCP has made the diagnosis of these anomalies relatively easy and has undoubtedly enabled clinicians to familiarize themselves with these pathologies. This has led to a considerable improvement in the therapeutic management of these malformations.

This work aims to review all medical aspects (the epidemiological, anatomopathological, clinical, morphological and therapeutic aspects) of the bilio-pancreatic malformations in adults.

LIST OF ABBREVIATIONS

CBD: Common Bile Duct
CDBD: Cystic Dilation of Bile Ducts
ERCP: Endoscopic Retrograde Cholangio-Pancreatography
ESM: Endoscopic Sphincterotomy of the Major Papilla
ESm: Endoscopic Sphincterotomy of the Minor Papilla
EUS: Endoscopic Ultrasound
IPMNP: Intra Papillary Mucinous Neoplasm of the Pancreas
MRCP: Magnetic Resonance Cholangio-Pancreatography
PBMJ: Pancreatico-biliary Maljunction
PDiv: Pancreas Divisum
S-MRCP: MRCP with Secretine Injection
SPPNP: Solid Pseudo Papillary Neoplasm of the Pancrea
US: Ultrasound

PART 1

CYSTIC DILATION OF BILE DUCTS & PANCREATICO-BILIARY MALJUNCTION

CHAPTER 1

INTRODUCTION

Cystic dilatations of the bile ducts (CDBD) are a rare congenital biliary malformation. It is defined as an ectasia of a part or all of the intra and/or extra hepatic bile ducts (1,2). It is worth noting that it must not be secondary to a tumor, a lithiasis or a biliary inflammation.

CDBD is frequently associated with a pancreatico-biliary maljunction (PBMJ). The incidence of CDBD varies from 1/100,000 to 1/150,000 in Western countries and is about 1/13,000 in some parts of Asia (3).

The most commonly used classification is that of Todani (3), which groups CDBD into five types according to the location, extent and type of dilatation of the bile ducts. The type I is the most common (80%) (6).

CDBD can be discovered during childhood but can remain asymptomatic for a very long time (4). Patients with CDBD may also develop several complications such as biliary lithiasis, acute cholangitis, acute pancreatitis, cyst rupture and the redoubtable cholangiocarcinoma of which risk is significantly higher than that of the general population (7).

The diagnosis of CDBD has been revolutionized by the advent of Magnetic Resonance Cholangio-pancreatography (MRCP) as it not only determines the type of CDBD according to the Todani classification but also allows to search for a PBMJ. Furthermore, this imaging may reveal a possible biliary degeneration. That is why MRCP is currently essential to guide the surgical attitude.

CHAPTER 2

HISTORY

In 1723, Vater conducted a study that described the normal anatomy and the anomalies of the bile ducts (8). Nevertheless, the first complete description of CDBD was reported by Gouglas in 1852 (9).

From the year 1920 onwards, numerous works were focused on this subject in order to propose etiopathogenic and/or therapeutic concepts: these are the studies of Zinniger and Cash (1932), Poate (1936), Tsoudakas and Robinette (1956) and Yotuyanagi (1936). The latter suggested the congenital origin of CDBD based on the theory of the inequality of epithelial proliferation (10-12).

In 1959, Caroli considered that CDBD is secondary to congenital atresia most often located at the bilio duodenal junction (13). This was subsequently refuted by Babitt in 1973, as he incriminated a biliopancreatic junction anomaly (anomaly of the biliary and pancreatic ducts fusion) defined by a combination of 3 criteria (5,14,15):

- A common channel over 15mm long.
- An extra duodenal junction of the two channels away from the sphincter.
- A connection angle greater than 30°.

Alonso-Lej proposed in 1959 the first classification of the choledochal cyst. It solely takes into account the cystic dilatation of extra hepatic bile ducts, and it was only in 1975 that the cystic dilatation of intra hepatic bile ducts was included in the classification by Flangian (16,17).

Finally, it was in 1977 that Todani drew up a complete classification of CDBD into 5 groups according to their morphological aspects (18,19).

CHAPTER 3

EPIDEMIOLOGY

1. Frequency

The CDBD is a rare congenital biliary pathology and still less frequent than biliary atresia (20). Its incidence is 1/13500 births in the United States, 1/15000 births in Australia, and Western countries (in general). It is remarkably more frequent in Asian populations with an incidence of 1/1000 births: it is worth noting that the two thirds of cases occur in Japan and only 0.3% are observed in South Korea (21).

2. Sex-Ratio

A clear female predominance is reported by all authors (22). The CDBD is encountered three times more often among women than men, with a sex ratio ranging from 1/4 to 1/3 (23,24).

3. Age

The CDBD affects all age ranges, but it is generally discovered in children, teenagers and young adults (25,26):

- Twenty-five percent (25%) of cases are infants under one-year-old.
- Sixty percent (60%) of cases are children under 10-year-old.
- Twenty percent (20%) of cases are diagnosed in adulthood (27, 28).
- Less than 1% of CDBD are diagnosed in patients over 70 years. To date, the extreme age of diagnosis is 87 years (29).

Currently, it is widely accepted that the CDBD is of congenital origin as many cases were discovered on antenatal ultrasound (from the 15th week of pregnancy).

Adult forms are generally CDBD that already exists since childhood but remained unnoticed because there were no symptoms (30).

CHAPTER 4

CLASSIFICATION OF CDBD

Alonso-Lej and his colleagues proposed the first CDBD classification in 1959. Then, Todani et al. reported in 1977 the most widely accepted classification, derived from Alonso-Lej's original classification and based on the site of cystic dilatation (31).

1. Todani classification

In 1977, Todani and his colleagues extended the [1st] classification of Alonso-Lej et al. made in 1959 (it included 3 types of CDBD).

The Todani's classification is typically morphological and takes into account both intra and extra hepatic bile ducts dilatations. It is currently, the most widely used classification (32).

1.1. Type I

It accounts for almost 90% of CDBD. The anomaly develops on the extra-hepatic bile duct below the intra-hepatic bile ducts and above the intra pancreatic portion of the choledocus.

A type I cyst may be associated with a slight dilation (or hypertrophy) of the intra-hepatic bile ducts secondary to biliary stasis. In addition, the cyst volume is variable and may hold more than one liter of bile.

There are 3 subtypes of Todani Type I CDBD. This differentiation is based on the location of the gallbladder in relation to the cyst on the one hand and on the dilation shape on the other hand (25) (Figure 4-1):

- *Type Ia:* it is a sacciform cystic dilation of the entire extra-hepatic common bile duct without intra-hepatic bile ducts involvement. The cystic duct (of the gallbladder) fits into the dilated duct.
- *Type Ib:* it is an isolated segmental dilation of the distal part of the common bile duct. The rest of the biliary tree is generally very normal.
- *Type Ic:* it is a smooth fusiform dilation of the common bile duct associated with a PBMJ (33).

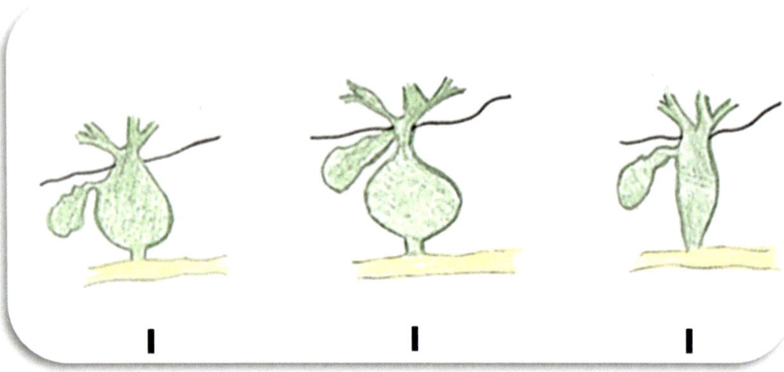

Figure 4-1: The 3 subgroups of CDBD type I according to the Todani classification. Type Ia: sacciform dilation. Type Ib: segmental dilatation. Type Ic: fusiform dilatation.

1.2. Type II

The type II of CDBD (2%) is a real diverticulum of the common bile duct. In general, it is a lateral sacciform dilation attached by a usually short and narrow pedicle to a non-cystic common bile duct (20). Such a diverticulum may resemble a duplication of the gallbladder.

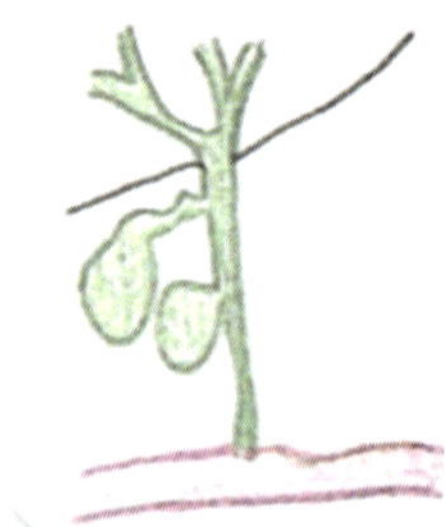

Figure 4-2: The type II of CDBD according to the Todani classification

1.3. Type III

The type III of CDBD, also called choledochocele, was reported for the first time by Wheeler in 1940. It is a cystic dilatation of the terminal portion of the common bile duct protruding into the duodenal lumen. The overlying portion of the common bile duct is usually normal or dilated but not cystic (34-37).

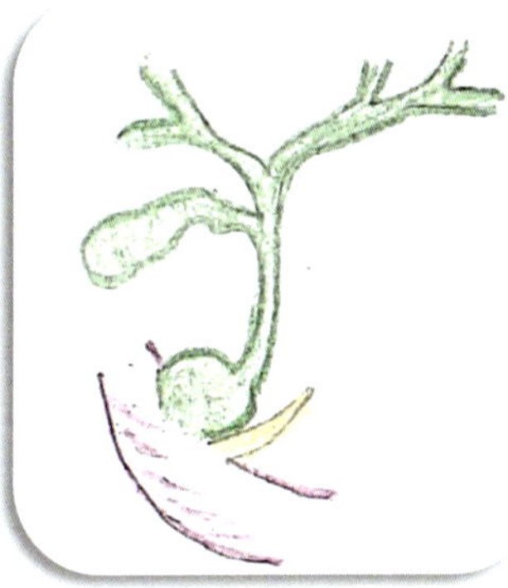

Figure 4-3: The type III of CDBD according to the Todani classification

1.4. Type IV

The type IV of CDBD may involve dilatation of both intra- and extra-hepatic bile ducts. They are classified into two subgroups, namely types IVA and IVB (38-41) (Figure 4-4):

- The type IVA: it is a cystic dilatation of the common bile duct, whatever its type, associated with intra-hepatic bile ducts cystic dilatation. The Intra-hepatic biliary dilatation is most often bi-lobar. When it is an associated uni-lobar dilation of intra-hepatic bile ducts, it is more frequently located in the left liver lobe.
- The type IVB: it is a multiple cystic dilatation of the extra-hepatic bile ducts, which may combine several of the previous types of CDBD. So, this type consists of multiple dilations of the common bile duct, classically described as a "string of pearls".

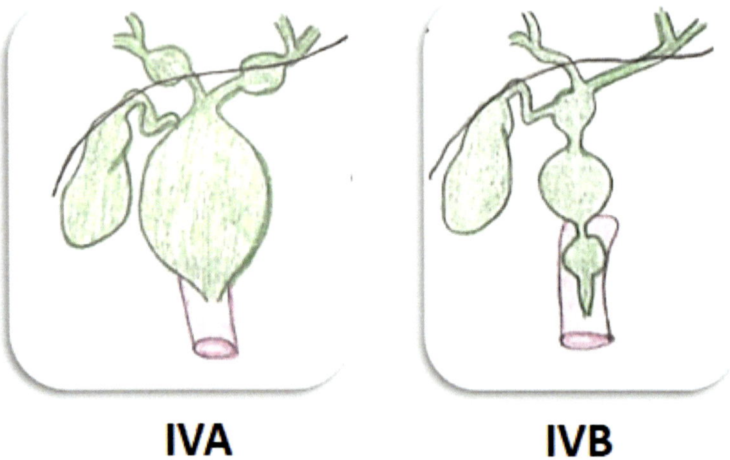

Figure 4-4: The type IV of CDBD according to the Todani classification

1.5. Type V

The type V of CDBD, also called Caroli disease, is a congenital, saccular or fusiform, non-obstructive dilatation of the intra hepatic bile ducts (42, 43).

In this case there may be intra hepatic biliary dilations interspersed with healthy ductular areas. This is called a rosary-like aspect of the intra hepatic biliary tree. They can be diffuse or localized and are most common in the left liver lobe. The extra-hepatic bile ducts can be normal or pathological. There are 2 subgroups of this kind (type V) of CDBD *(44)*:

- *The 1st subgroup or type I or Caroli disease:* it is a pure form of the CDBD type IV. The liver is apparently normal and there is no congenital hepatic fibrosis. This form concerns young adults (< 30 years) and the occurrence of acute cholangitis is common.
- *The 2nd subgroup or type II or Caroli syndrome:* it is a mixed form of the CDBD type IV. There is a congenital hepatic fibrosis with a bulky and harsh liver. The size and morphology of the dilated intra-hepatic bile ducts are variable (44).

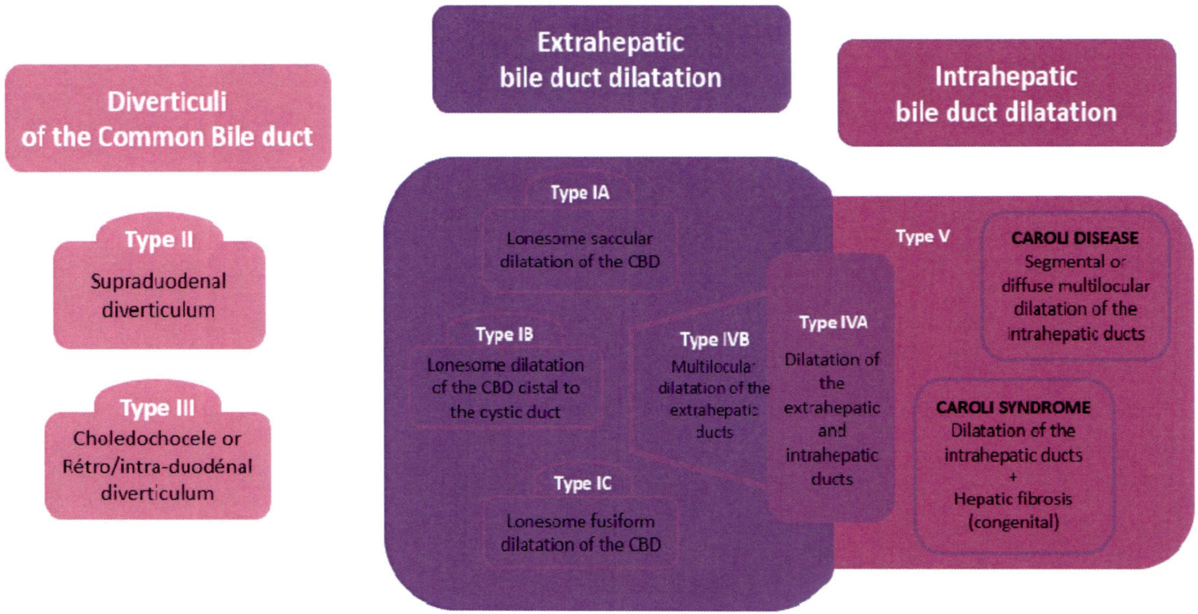

Figure 4-5: Diagram showing the morphological characteristics of bile ducts that Todani's classification is based on.

Both subgroups of this CDBD type V may be associated with the "Autosomal Recessive Polycystic Kidney Disease" known as ARPKD (26, 43). In this case, the CDBD is considered to be a ductal plaque malformation at different levels of intra hepatic bile ducts leading to varying degrees of biliary dilatation. In addition, this condition is associated to a periportal fibrosis that is a decisive element not only for the diagnosis of this CDBD Type V but also for ruling out differential diagnoses (17, 45, 46).

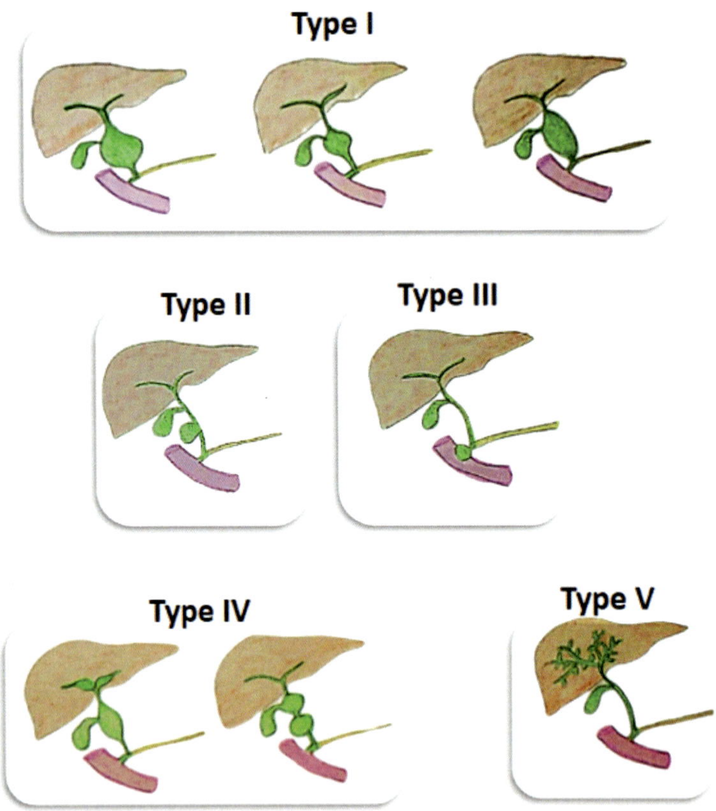

Figure 4-6: Todani classification of CDBD

The table 4-1 shows the proportions of CDBD types in Mediterranean and North African series.

Table 4-1: Percentage of CDBD types (according to the Todani classification) in different North African series.

Study	Country	Year	Type of CDBD				
			I	II	III	IV	V
Mannai S. et al. (47)	Tunisia	2006	61,1%	0%	0%	0%	38,8%
Dry F. et al. (48)	Morocco - Fez	2014	33,3%	0%	0%	55%	0%
Erraoui G. et al. (34)	Morocco Marrakech	2018	66,6%	0%	0%	33,3%	0%

1.6. New Type VI

Actually, there is no type VI in Todani's classification. However, several publications reported a new type of CDBD affecting the cystic duct alone or in association with another type of CDBD. Indeed, isolated dilatation of the cystic duct is not part of any of the 5 types of the Todani classification. This is why several authors suggested to add this anomaly as Todani type VI or as a subgroup of Todani type II (40, 49).
It is worth noting that differentiation between type VI and type II CDBD may not be easy on preoperative imaging (40).
Furthermore, in some cases, cystic duct dilatation that wraps around the CBD can lead to dilatation of the upstream bile ducts and would cause confusion with the type IVA on preoperative imaging. In this case, intraoperative exploration remains the only way to distinguish between the two types (49).
Ackermann T et al. (50) even suggest subdividing type VI into 2 subgroups:

- The VIA type: isolated cyst of the cystic duct.
- The VIB type: cystic dilatation or cyst of the cystic duct associated with CBD dilatation.

From another point of view, this type VI can be subdivided into fusiform (more common) or saccular subgroups according to Amarjothi JMV et al. (51).

2. Other classifications

2.1. Visser Classification

Visser and colleagues (44, 52) believe that the distinction between CDBD types I and IVA is arbitrary, since there is usually some impairment of the intrahepatic channels in both classes. They further argue that gallbladder-like diverticulum, choledococele and Caroli's disease are unrelated to CDBD. Therefore, they suggest to use a descriptive terminology instead of Todani's classification (Figure 4-7).

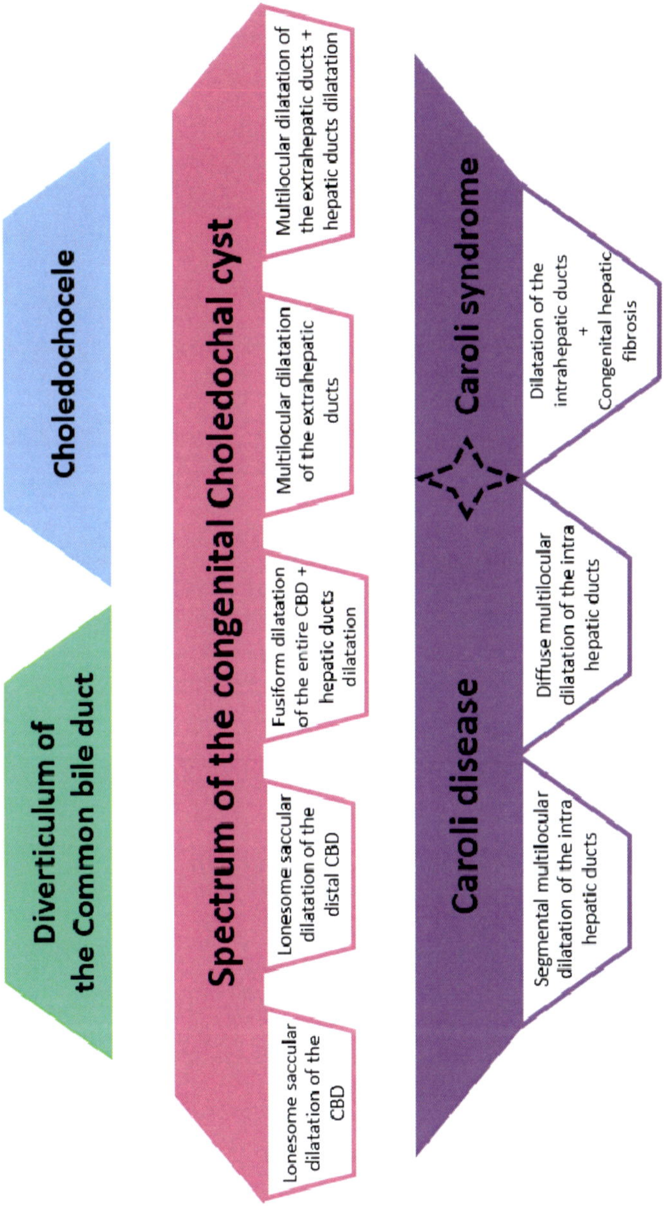

Figure 4-7: Visser's classification (descriptive terminology) of CDBD based on pathophysiological criteria.

Lilly et al. described an entity called the "crude form", in which patients have PBMJ and typical CDBD symptoms without any dilatation of the bile ducts. Sarin et al. believe that this form should be included in the CDBD spectrum (53).

Kaneyama et al. reported 4 cases of type II diverticulum as a consequence of CDBD type IC. This anomaly was described as a mixed CDBD type (I and II) (54). This represents 1.1% of cases in their series of 356 patients.

2.2. Modified Todani classification

Kronfli R et al. (55) proposed to update the Todani classification by modifying the types IV and I (Figure 4-8). This proposal stems from their study comparing pressures and amylase levels in bile duct cysts in these two types of CDBD. This modification mainly targets type IV, but it systematically leads to a change in the type I subgroups.

Thus, type IV is subdivided into:

- *IVF:* fusiform choledochal cyst with a relatively low intra-cystic pressure and high levels of bile amylase. In this case, patients are generally older at the time of surgery.
- *IVC:* saccular choledochal cyst with relatively high intra-cystic pressure and low bile amylase levels. In this case, patients are relatively *younger* at the time of surgery.

This is a subdivision based on clinical and morphological criteria.

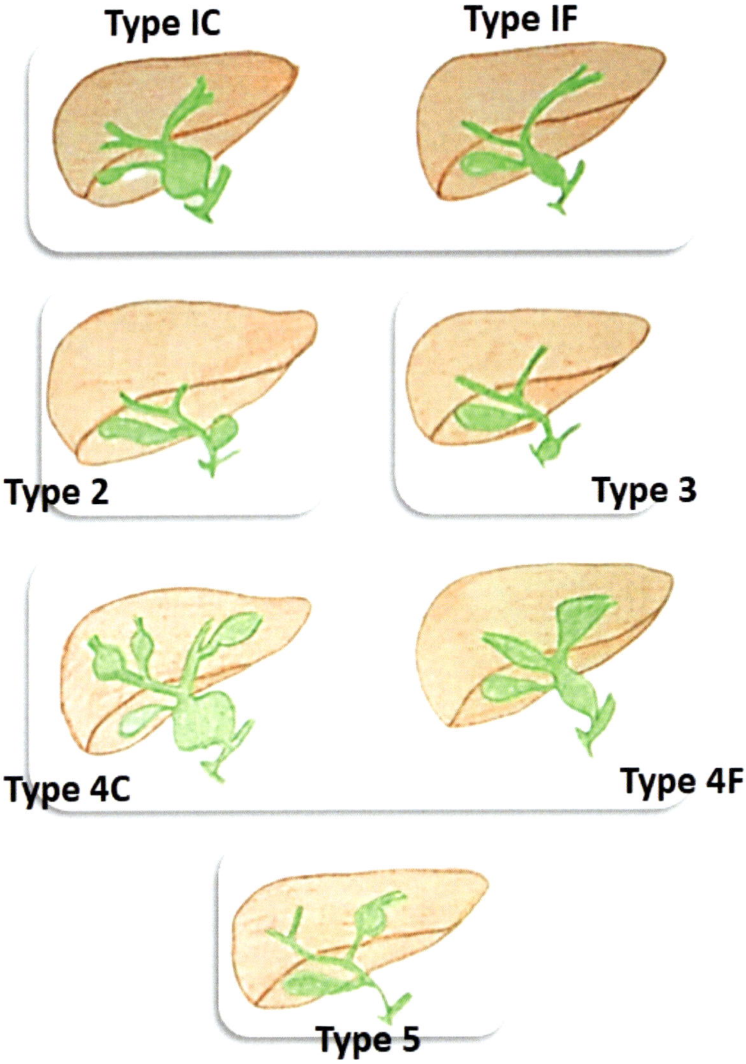

Figure 4-8: Modified Todani classification proposed by Kronfli R et al.

CHAPTER 5

PANCREATICO-BILIARY MALJUNCTION (PBMJ)

1. Definition of PBMJ

Normally, the bile duct and the Wirsung canal drain into the duodenum through the major papilla in two ways: either separately, or in 65-90% of cases, through a common channel whose average length is 4.6 +/- 2.6mm in adults.

Nowadays, it is well established that CDBD is the consequence of a PBMJ according to Babbit's theory (56), however this does not explain CDBD without PBMJ. This is why other etiologies have been suggested such as viral cause and defective nerve supply of bile ducts. In addition, some authors suggested an embryological hypothesis stating that PBMJ is linked to the pancreatic ventral bud malrotation. The fusion of the two (ventral and dorsal) pancreatic buds could be done in an oblique position that leads to the formation of a long common channel (57).

This anomaly is found in 70% and 30% of cases respectively of Todani type Ia and Ic CDBD (58).

The old definition of the PBMJ is based on several anatomopathological criteria (58):

- *A major criterion:* a common biliopancreatic channel which length is greater than 10mm in adults. It is known as the "long common channel".
- *Two minor criteria:*
  - Extra duodenal junction upstream of the Oddi sphincter of the biliary and pancreatic ducts.
  - Bilio-pancreatic connection angle greater than 30°.

However, the PBMJ is currently defined, according to the new Japanese recommendations of 2015, as a biliopancreatic junction located outside the duodenal wall. This should be revealed by imaging and possibly confirmed by histological examination (56-58). The presence of CDBD or a high level of bile amylases are two other secondary but not mandatory criteria for the diagnosis of PBMJ.

The common biliopancreatic channel may induce chronic pancreatic-biliary reflux. Therefore, noting the considerable increase in the concentration of amylases in samples of bile taken from the CBD upstream of this common channel, some authors have decided to add this biochemical criterion to the definition of PBMJ.

2. Classifications of PBMJ

2.1. Komi classification

Komi et al. (34, 59) proposed a classification of PBMJ, based on 2 criteria:

- The bilio-pancreatic junction angle (between the pancreatic duct and the CBD).
- A long common channel.

This classification has a dual purpose as it has therapeutic implications and prognostic interest.
According to this Komi classification, there are 3 types of PBMJ (Figure 5-1):

- *Type I:* known also as "Wirsung in choledocus" or "W in C".
  - Ia: PBMJ without CDBD.
  - Ib: PBMJ with CDBD.
- *Type II:* known also as "Choledocus in Wirsung" or "C in W".
  - IIa: PBMJ without CDBD.
  - IIb: PBMJ with CDBD.
- *Type III:* in addition to the PBMJ, there is an associated accessory pancreatic duct, connected or not to the biliary and pancreatic ducts.

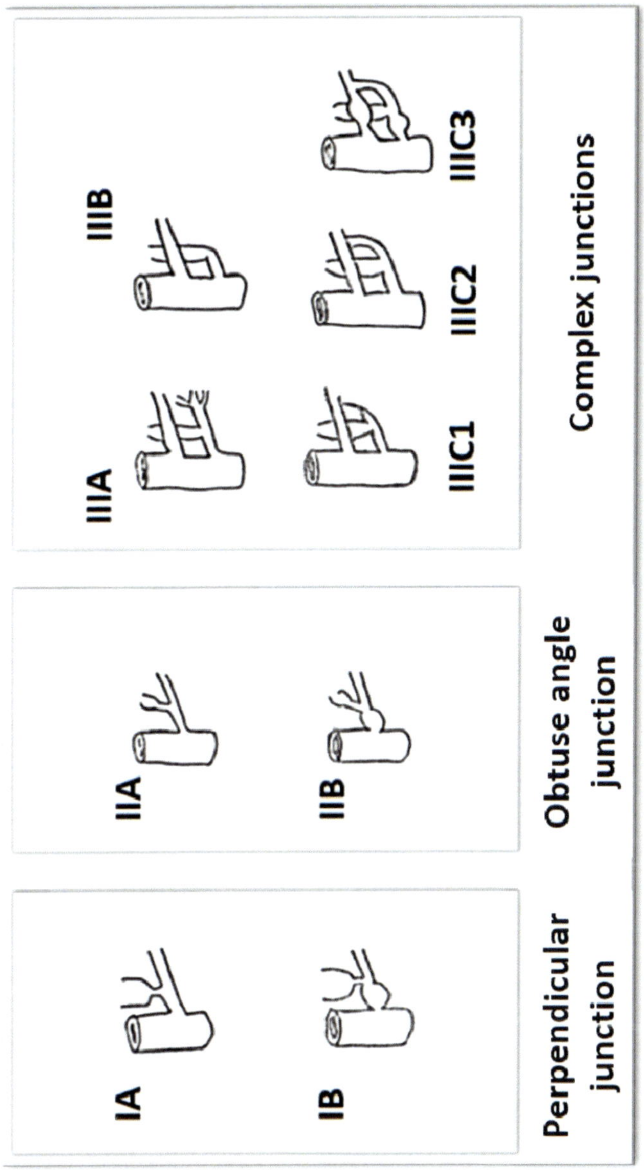

Figure 5-1: Komi classification of AJBPs.

2.2. Kimura classification

Kimura et al. suggested to classify the PBMJ in two varieties (34):

- *Type 1:* the pancreatic excretory canal seems to be flowing into the bile duct.
- *Type 2:* this is more common. In this type, the bile duct seems to flow into the Wirsung.

Thus, this classification seems less elaborate than that of Komi.

2.3. Japanese classification of 2015

This is the JSPBM ("Japanese Study Group of Pancreato-biliary Maljunction") classification published in 2015 as shown in Figure 5-2 (56).

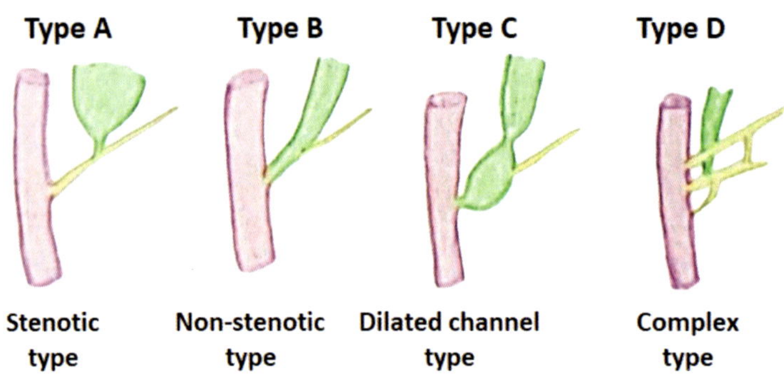

Figure 5-2: Japan's 2015 BPA classification.

CHAPTER 6

ANATOMOPATHOLOGICAL STUDY

1. Macroscopic study

1.1. Volume of choledochal cyst

Some authors studied the vertical and transverse diameters of the choledochal cyst, while other authors appreciated the amount of fluid contained in the cyst. However, it is usual to find a voluminous biliary cystic dilatation.

The smallest case reported in the literature (1910) measures 2.5cm wide and 3cm long. The largest CDBD containing 8 liters of bile, was reported by Red and Rubd in 1922 (57, 58).

1.2. Choledochal cyst wall

The wall of the cystic portions of the bile ducts has a very variable appearance: it may be pale and crossed by a more or less dense vascular network, and sometimes it may be bluish and slightly vascularized. This aspect variation is related to the thickness of the CDBD wall. Indeed, this wall is usually thick (it may reach 1cm) but sometimes it may be very thin, hence the risk of rupture particularly during surgery (34).

The fibrosis-like aspect of the cyst wall, which is lined with columnar epithelium and the site of lymphocyte infiltration, is typical in pediatric CDBD (59).

1.3. Choledochal cyst contents

The content of the choledochal cyst is usually a bile of varying color and consistency. This bile can be either aseptic or most often infected, depending on the degree of obstruction in the bottom of the common bile duct.

In addition, parietal calcifications as well as intra cystic calculi can be found in about 20% of cases (59).

2. Microscopic study

The cystic wall is made up of sclerotic connective tissue, within which there are a few rare elastic fibers and muscle cells. It is lined with an almost destroyed epithelium of the squamous biliary type. In fact, this epithelium is generally made up of a few areas of flattened or cubic, inflammatory and ulcerated cells. It is also covered with a fibrino-leukocyte coating, and it has a basal connective condensation (60).

In adults, the CDBD wall has signs of inflammation and hyperplasia. The common findings of histological examination of all types of CDBD show acute and/or chronic mucosal inflammation, mucosal dysplasia and few (or no) mucus-producing glands (59).

Furthermore, microscopic study of the CDBD wall has shown that there are two histological types:

- A glandular form: there is dilations of the mucous membrane glands and more or less intense inflammation. It is usually associated with BPMJ.
- A fibrous form: with circumferential thickening of the low inflammatory CDBD wall. It is less often associated with PBMJ.

The bile contained in the CDBD is frequently superinfected with gram-negative germs.

Degeneration to adenocarcinoma is possible and has been most frequently reported in Japan (61).

The theory suggested by many authors states that the intercellular space of the biliary epithelial junction is rapidly damaged as soon as it is exposed to pancreatic juice. The mucous barrier of the bile duct is made up of mucus at the surface cell epithelium. Once this barrier is destroyed, inflammation sets in, followed by degeneration of the elastic fibers and proliferation of collagen fibers. Then there will be a significant defect of the biliary epithelium leading to subsequent cystic dilatation of the bile ducts. This hypothesis was later confirmed by studies which showed that the effects of pancreatic reflux in the common bile duct to be responsible of CDBD (59).

CHAPTER 7

CLINICAL PRESENTATION

1. Circumstances of CDBD discovery

Most CDBD are diagnosed in childhood. Nevertheless, it may be discovered in adulthood (approximately 25% of cases) (7).

The classic clinical presentation of CDBD is the BERNHEIM's clinical triad, which combines a palpable mass of the right hypochondrium, jaundice and pain in the same hypochondrium. However, this triad would only be present in 6 to 20% of cases (30, 31) because patients would generally have one or two symptoms of this triad. Moreover, it should be noted that most cases of CDBD are revealed by only one of these three clinical signs (32).

2. Clinical manifestations

CDBD is usually diagnosed in childhood (75%) but it has atypical clinical presentation in adults as the symptoms become less discernible. Indeed, the classic clinical triad (abdominal pain, jaundice and right hypochondrium mass) is frequently seen in pediatric patients whereas adults are more likely to be asymptomatic or have only abdominal pain. Cystic dilation and distal stenoses result in chronic inflammation, biliary stasis (with liver enzymes high levels) and stone formation leading to complications such as jaundice, pancreatitis, cholangitis, portal hypertension (62, 63).

2.1. Abdominal pain

This is the main clinical sign of CDBD. Indeed almost 60% of patients may present with abdominal pain, and it is the most frequent symptom in adults (97% of cases) (58).

The pain is related to the hyper pressure in the bile ducts due to the latent obstacle. Its usual site is the right hypochondrium, but sometimes it may be a generalized abdominal pain. More rarely, it may be located in the epigastrium or in the peri-umbilical region (58, 59).

The pain may irradiate towards the right thorax base or to the right shoulder. The pain intensity and rhythmicity are very variable: it is sometimes paroxysmal and violent, as a real hepatic colic, and sometimes it is a dull but not very intense pain. It may also be a simple abdominal discomfort. Other pain types were also reported, such as cramps, twisting or even burning. Associated signs may also be noticed mainly nausea and vomiting (34).

2.2. Jaundice

It is a sign of great importance that points to a liver or to a biliary tract disorder. Jaundice is of variable frequency and intensity, and is the most frequent CDBD discovery circumstance in children (70% of cases), whereas in adults its frequency is only 50%. It is worth noting that 77% of patients would present with retentional jaundice: dark urine and discolored stools with possible pruritus of variable ferocity (34, 64).

The jaundice is related to a more or less significant biliary obstruction caused by the rebounding of the cyst's bottom, which attracts and bends the lower part of the common bile duct.

Jaundice may present with many forms (48):

- *Sub-icterus* that can go unnoticed.
- *Acute cholangitis:* straightforward and painful jaundice associated with a feverish state. Physical examination may reveal a hepatomegaly.
- *Variable or fluctuating jaundice:* suggesting a CBD lithiasis.
- Progressive *neoplastic-type jaundice.*

2.3. Right hypochondrium mass

It is a painless, smooth, regular, soft renitent and well limited right hypochondrium mass.

Its incidence decreases with age, ranging from 65% in subjects under 10 years to 30% in patients aged between 10 and 30 years. In addition, only 9.8% of patients over 30-year-old would have such a mass (36).

The volume of this mass is variable:

- It can be huge (2 liters), distending the abdomen, descending below the umbilicus and extending beyond the midline.
- The volume of this mass is sometimes variable in the same patient, reflecting the occasional filling and emptying of the cystic pouch.

It is worth noting that this mass can be sometimes mistaken for hepatomegaly.

2.4. Other clinical signs

Besides this triad, other symptoms can be reported:

- *Fever:* frequent but not specific. It is related to a biliary infection and can take several forms:
  - Isolated fever (approximately at 38° C).
  - Acute cholangitis (fever at 38°-39° C), often accompanied by chills, bilious vomiting and jaundice.

Its frequency varies from 10% to 61.3% according to the several publications (43.44).

- *Hepatomegaly:* this is a large cholestatic liver observed in 7.5% of cases (46).
- *Signs of portal hypertension:* these are only seen in case of associated congenital liver fibrosis.
- *Other general signs:* weight loss and general_condition alteration.
- *Functional signs:*
  - Vomiting is sometimes the only or the first symptom. It may be bilious or a very abundant food vomiting. It is related to a heavy reflux of bile from the cyst into the duodenum (43, 48).
  - Dark urine and discolored stools are part of retentional jaundice (49).

2.5. Main complications

CDBD can often remain asymptomatic. However, it may be rarely discovered when a complication occurs such as biliary perforation, biliary and hepatic infection, acute pancreatitis, cirrhosis with portal hypertension and malignant degeneration.

The complications' frequency increases with age of the patient. Indeed, they were reported in 0.7% of subjects under 10 years and in 6.8% of patients between 11 and 20-year-old but they are much more frequent in adults (30, 34, 65).

CHAPTER 8

BIOLOGICAL FINDINGS

They are of no diagnostic interest since they have no specificity (66). The biological assessment may be strictly normal. However, it would help to objectify infection, cholestasis and alteration of liver function.

1. Blood count

It reveals hyperleukocytosis mainly made of polynuclear cells, which indicate infection of the bile ducts (38).

2. Liver tests

Various disturbances of the liver function tests can be observed (67) such as cholestasis, hepatic cytolysis (high transaminase levels are generally lower than those found in the bile ducts congenital atresia) and hepatic insufficiency. The lowering of prothrombin levels and the decrease in cholesterol esterification settle late and reflect hepatic sclerosis. This leads to cirrhosis, which has a poor prognosis.

3. Pancreatic enzymes assay

Whether there is acute pancreatitis or not, hyper-amylasemia can be observed in 35% of cases in adults (54), whereas in children it remains exceptional (55).

Several recent publications have reported the association of CDBD with PBMJ in about 90-100% of cases, and a high concentration of pancreatic enzymes in the bile ducts (55). When common bile duct pressure increases due to obstructive cholangitis, pancreatic enzymes in the bile can pass into the blood-stream. This means that cholangio-venous amylase reflux would probably cause a hyper-amylasemia (68, 69).

CHAPTER 9

IMAGERY

The morphological assessment plays a crucial role in the diagnosis of CDBD.

1. Abdominal Ultrasound

The first CDBD diagnosed by ultrasound was reported by GILDAY in 1969.

It is a safe, non-invasive, easy, simple to perform and reliable examination in assessing the extent of bile ducts dilatation. It has become the first-line examination (69, 70) performed in almost all patients with hepatobiliary symptoms. Its diagnostic reliability varies from 85 to 100% of cases (61).

It also allows an antenatal diagnosis of CDBD from 15 weeks of pregnancy onwards (48).

The cyst appears as an oval, anechoic, posteriorly enhanced (acoustic enhancement) mass with a fluid-filled structure that may contain stones (63). US also allows to explore the liver and the rest of the biliary ducts (64).

In general, US diagnosis of CDBD is easy, particularly for non-bulky cysts, with no obvious calculous or tumor obstacle (71).

According to the new recommendations of the Japanese Society of Hepato-biliopancreatic Surgery published in May 2016, the internal diameter of the most dilated site of the common bile duct should be considered as the maximum diameter of CDBD. Since the standard diameter of CBD measured by ultrasound is significantly correlated with age, the diagnosis of dilatation is based on the upper limit of CBD diameter in each patient (72).

Ultrasound monitoring of these cysts allows early detection of possible degeneration into cholangiocarcinoma. This will be suspected if the US examination reveals a thickening and/or irregularity of the cystic wall.

US images are sometimes difficult to interpret, especially in patients with history of previous biliary surgery or in case of any inflammation of the liver pedicle (27).

2. Abdominal CT-Scan

It provides little additional information compared to abdominal US with regard to the exploration of the bile ducts (72).

The CT-scan shows the CDBD as a very limited hypodense fluid structure between the hepatic hilum and the duodenum possibly associated to a biliary lithiasis. It allows a better study of the hepatic parenchyma and would help for intra hepatic bile ducts' evaluation (71) .

CT scans are also helpful in the differential diagnosis between Caroli disease and polycystic liver disease (72).

The Cholangio-scan is a specific imagery technique for the visualization of the bile ducts by injecting an intravenous biliary excretion contrast medium. A cartography of the biliary tree and a precise delimitation of the lesion are then obtained thanks to sagittal or 3D coronal reconstructions (72-76).

As a general rule, this Cholangio-scan is performed out of context of a standard abdominal Ct-scan , in order to allow better detection of small bile calculi (in the absence of a biliary obstruction) or to visualize the bile ducts anatomy with possible variants before surgery (75).

The indication for Cholangio-scan still nowadays very limited because of two reasons: first, the side effects of biliary contrast medium intravenous injection are more frequent than those of standard contrast medium (that needs renal excretion) and second a good biliary excretory function is required for high quality images (76).

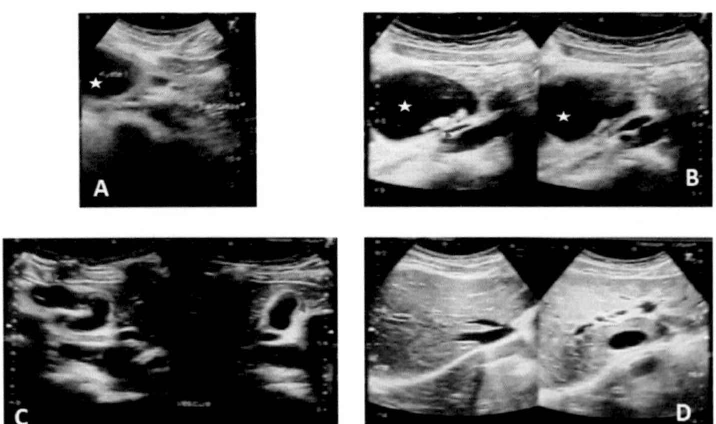

Figure 9-1: Abdominal ultrasound images showing a choledochal cyst (A and B: yellow star) containing bile sediments (pink arrow heads). There is also a slight dilation of the intra hepatic bile ducts (D). The gallbladder (red arrow heads) has a thin wall and doesn't contain any lithiasis (C).

3. Magnetic resonance cholangiopancreatography (MRCP)

This is the reference imaging modality allowing a careful exploration of the biliopancreatic ducts. It is a non-invasive and atraumatic technique (77, 78). However, it requires sometimes patient anesthesia or contrast medium injection.

The MRCP is very sensitive (70% to 100%) and specific (90% to 100%) in the diagnosis and classification of CDBD (79). Moreover, it allows reliable identification of PBMJ (particularly with secretin intravenous injection), as well as cholangiocarcinoma and biliary lithiasis 79-84).

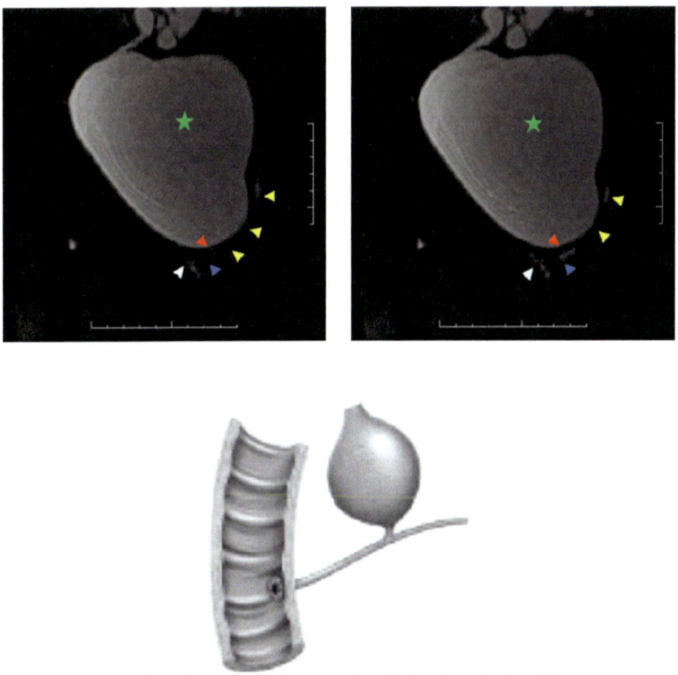

Figure 9-2: MRCP showing a PBMJ type Ia of the Komi classification and type A of the Japanese classification. Green asterisk: choledochal cyst. Yellow arrow head: Wirsung. Red arrow head: the distal fine (non-dilated) portion of the choledocus. Bule arrow head: the common channel.

It shows all biliary tree malformations and allow to differentiate CDBD from an obstructive pathology especially biliary one. In addition, it is very helpful in diagnosing biliary degeneration by showing a polyploid endoluminal tumor and/or a thickened irregular aspect of the biliary cystic wall.

The MRCP is an examination that can be performed on pregnant women in order to make an antenatal diagnosis of CDBD without mother or fetus radiation risks (59).

The principle of MRCP is the realization of very highly weighted T2 sequences (85), which wipe off the signal of both non-liquid structures and moving liquids, in order to show only the stagnant liquids' signal. In addition, it gives a hyper signal to long T2 tissues such as bile whereas it provides a hypo signal to shorter T2 tissues such as liver and pancreas. Vessels are hypo-signaling by magnetic phase shift (86).

The MRCP techniques consistently show the extra-hepatic bile ducts from the right and left hepatic ducts to the Vater ampulla as well as the pancreatic ducts (47, 87). The accessory biliary system including the gallbladder and the cystic duct is also visualized. In addition, real anatomical sections could be obtained by this imaging modality (88).

The MRCP performance in the diagnosis of bile and pancreatic ducts anatomical variants has been estimated as very high at approximately 98% (89).

Although MRCP is associated with lower morbidity (82), its ability to detect minor ductal abnormalities or small choledochal cyst remains relatively limited (90-97).

The MRI aspects of the most frequent types of CDBD according to Todani classification are illustrated in the tables 9-1 and 9-2 below.

Table 9-1: MRI aspects of the most frequent Todani types of CDBD (part 1)

CDBD type according to Todani classification		**Schematic illustration**	**MRCP aspect**
	A	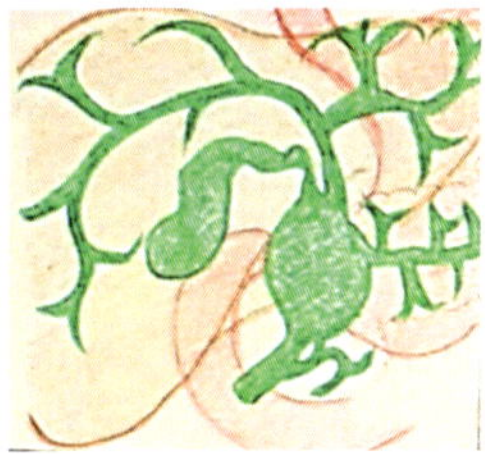	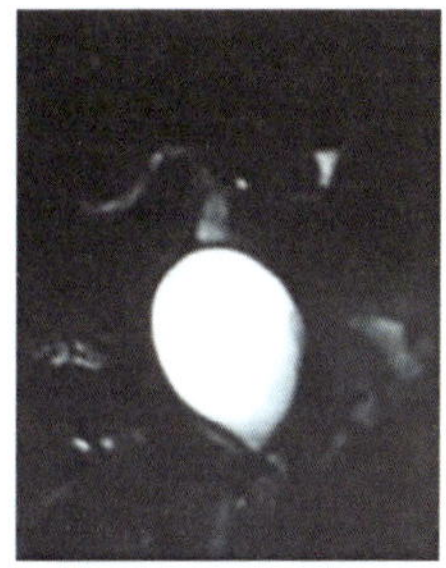
I (50-80%)	**B**	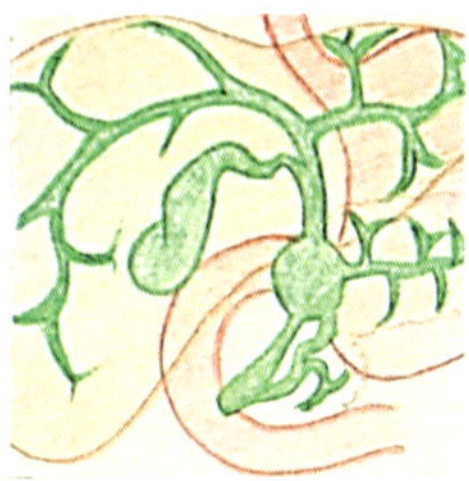	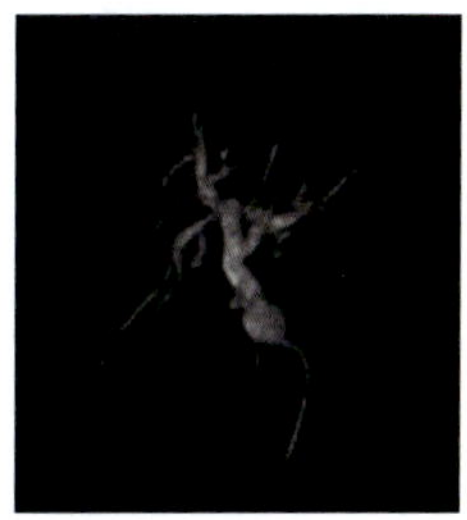
	C	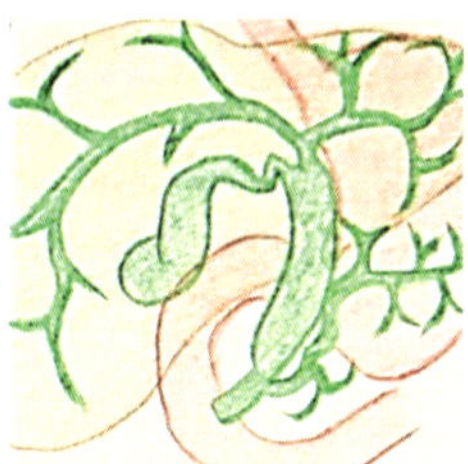	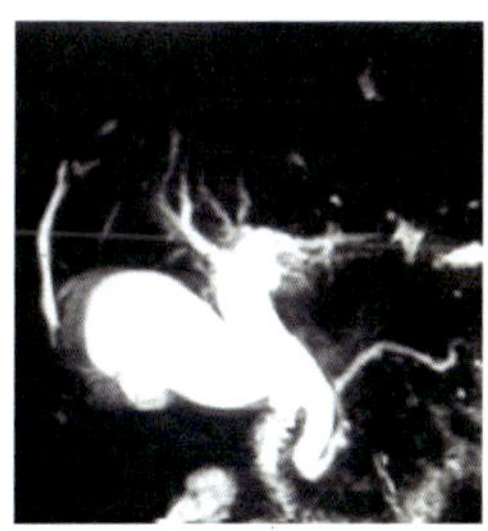

Table 9-2: MRI aspects of the most frequent Todani types of CDBD (part 2)

CDBD type according to Todani classification		Schematic illustration	MRCP aspect
IV (15-35%)	A	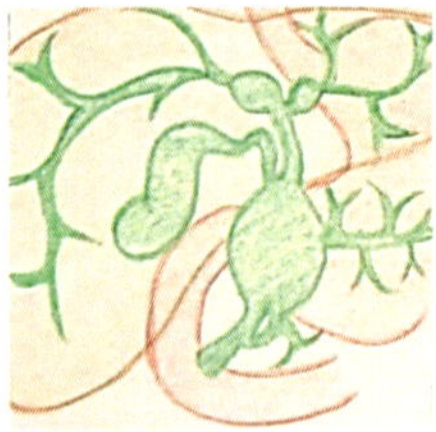	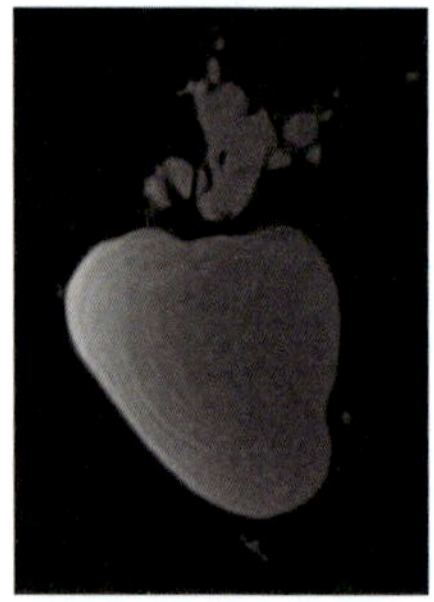
	B	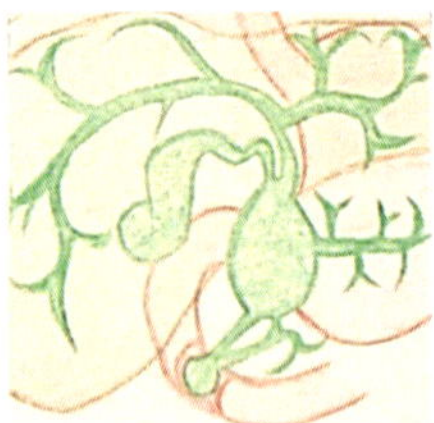	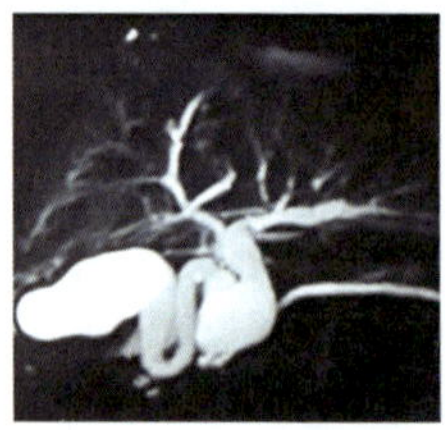
V (1%)		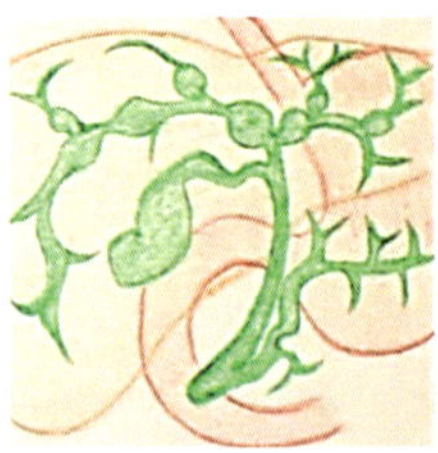	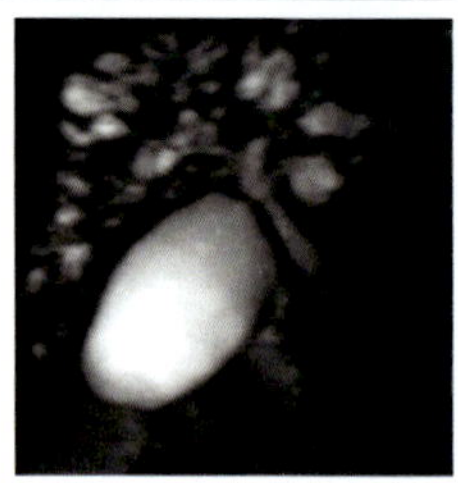

4. Bilio-Pancreatic Endoscopic Ultrasound

Its contribution has rarely been evaluated. Some studies have confirmed the excellent sensitivity of this imaging modality for:

- The diagnosis of choledochal cysts.
- The search and analysis of the variety of a PBMJ.
- Looking for arguments in favor of a possible associated tumor lesion, particularly vesicular one (98, 99).

5. Endoscopic Retrograde Cholangiopancreatography (ERCP)

It is one of the best techniques in the diagnosis and treatment of biliopancreatic disorders. One of its major roles is to give a precise image of pancreato-biliary duct abnormalities. It most often precedes an endoscopic therapeutic procedure (99, 100).

Although, ERCP is currently less commonly used for diagnostic purposes due to the performance of other diagnostic methods (CT-scan, CPRM and endoscopic ultrasound), it remains of specific interest for the diagnosis of early ductal lesions (e.g. sclerosing cholangitis and chronic pancreatitis), ductal anatomical variations (PBMJ, CDBD) and ampullary tumor pathology (100).

6. Percutaneous Transhepatic Cholangiography

It is a sensitive technique for defining the anatomy of the biliary tree, and it is particularly useful for the evaluation of intra hepatic biliary ducts.

It can be rarely performed preoperatively in case of jaundice for example. The percutaneous opacification of the dilated bile ducts is possible in the majority of cases.

A fine needle puncture is usually performed in the intra hepatic bile ducts under ultrasound or CT-scan control. However, this invasive imaging modality is rarely used in the context of CDBD (77). Moreover, it can sometimes be technically difficult and may require sometimes general anesthesia.

The percutaneous trans-hepatic cholangiography can cause some complications such as hemorrhage, choleperitoneum and superinfection. Thus, parenteral antibiotic prophylaxis and correction of a possible hemostasis disorder are recommended (77).

In addition, percutaneous cholangiography seems limited in the evaluation of the distal, intra-pancreatic and even intra-duodenal parts of the CBD (77).

In practice, this technique is reserved for situations in which MRCP or ERCP cannot be performed or are unable to visualize adequately the intra-hepatic ducts due to a proximal obstruction. However, these two conditions remain exceptional hence this imaging modality is currently being abandoned.

7. Biliary Scintigraphy

Technetium-99m biliary scintigraphy (trimethylindo-diacetic acid) is a simple, non-invasive and reproducible imaging method with good sensitivity for the morphological evaluation and classification of choledochal cyst. However, it has a lower sensitivity for the assessment of the intra-hepatic cystic bile ducts.

Nowadays, some physicians use biliary scintigraphy as part of the qualitative and quantitative functional analysis of the surgical procedures particularly bilio-digestive anastomosis.

This scintigraphy can show not only the CBD but also the intra-cystic cumulation of the radioactive product. In addition, it allows the study of liver function by assessing the capacity of the liver to fix iodine (34, 101).

8. Intraoperative Cholangiography

It perfectly shows the complete anatomy of the biliary and pancreatic ductal systems, but in some cases the distal bile duct is not opacified.

Its sensitivity varies from 92% to 96% and its specificity is almost 100%. It can be done either through the gallbladder (cystic duct) or by direct puncture of the cystic dilatation.

Cholangiography may be considered when the preoperative work-up does not provide sufficient information on the pancreato-biliary junction and/or the existence of a possible long common duct.

Intraoperative cholangiography offers the possibility of visualizing the intra hepatic biliary tree. This would help to detect a possible intra-hepatic biliary dilatation.

It also allows the surgeon to detect a possible biliary stenosis (34).

In practice, intraoperative cholangiography can show:

- The aspect of cystic dilatation of extra hepatic and/or intra hepatic bile ducts.
- The possible obstacle explaining this dilatation.
- And possibly the PBMJ if it exists.

The table 9-3 shows MRI aspect of some types of CDBD and the correspondent cholangiographic aspect.

Table 9-3*:* Aspects of certain types of CDBD on CPRM and intraoperative cholangiography

Todani type of CDBD	**MRCP aspect**	**Cholangiographic aspect**
Type IVa	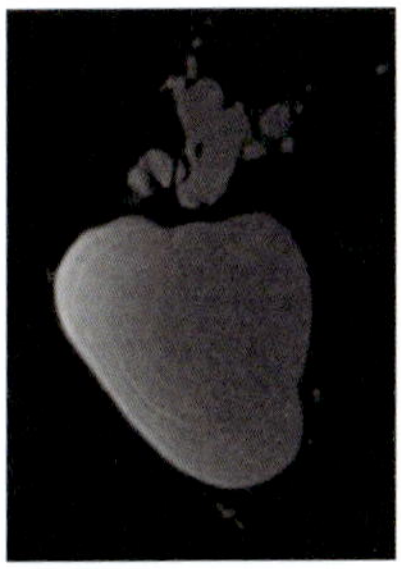	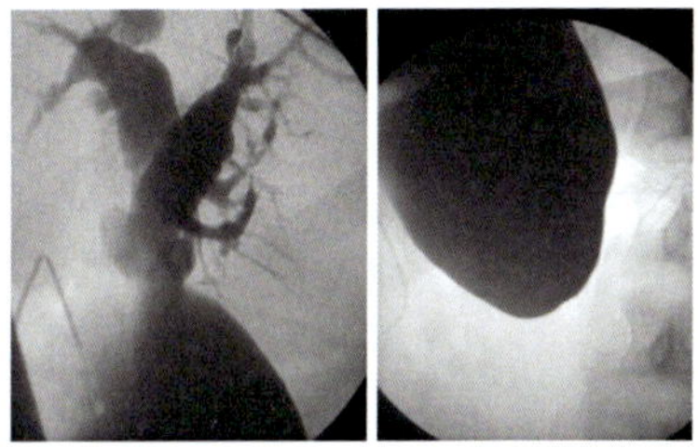
Type IVb	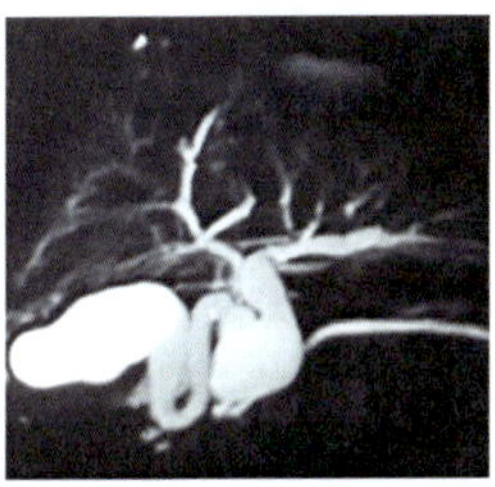	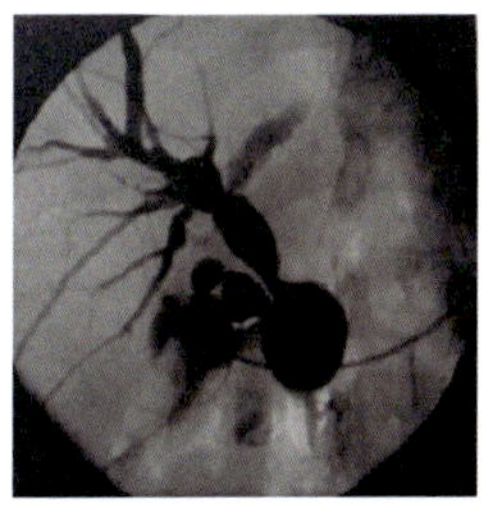
Type V	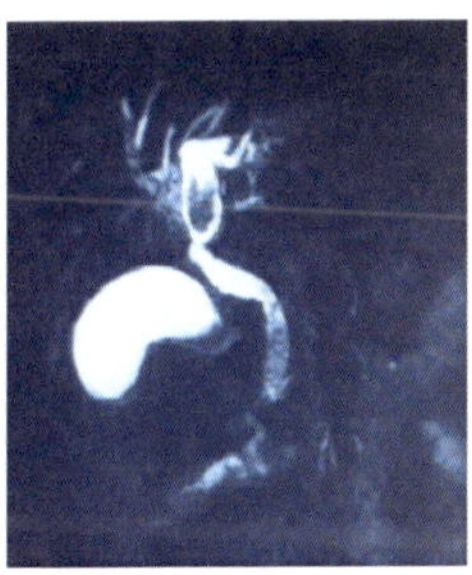	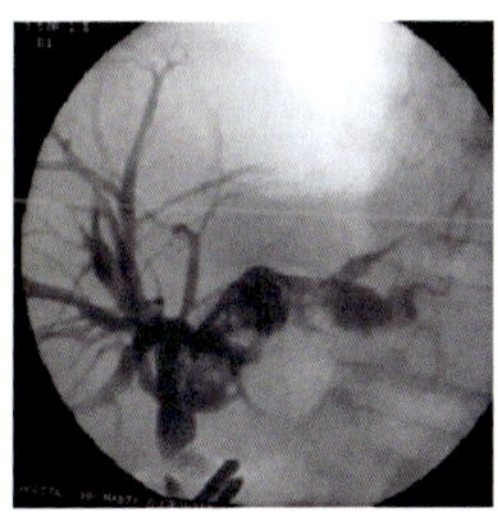
	Caroli disease: Cystic dilatation of left intra hepatic ducts with left intrahepatic lithiasis and choledochal stones	

CHAPTER 10

EVOLUTION AND COMPLICATIONS

The spontaneous evolution of CDBD is most often unfavorable as chronic cholestasis and infection can lead more or less rapidly to ascending cholangitis and secondary biliary cirrhosis with portal hypertension (15-32%).

In the absence of treatment, there is a high risk (5-17%) of cancerization of the cyst wall, which is the most serious and feared complication. The risk of degeneration increases to 100 times. The prognosis of such cholangiocarcinoma is very poor with an average overall survival of 8 months (84).

Other complications may occur such as (34):

- Biliary lithiasis (8-25%) which can block the lower bile duct,
- Cholangitis (11%) with possible septicemia or liver abscess,
- Cyst perforation with choleperitoneum or biliary peritonitis (3-7%), and
- Acute pancreatitis (0.5-33%).

1. Infectious Complications

1.1. Acute Cholangitis / Infection of Cyst Contents

It accounts for 11% of complications. It is mainly related to the biliary stasis and to the intra-cystic fluid infection. The most involved germs are the gram-negative bacilli. This acute cholangitis is a medical and surgical emergency.

Clinically, the cyst infection causes episodes of moderate fever, usually easily managed by antibiotherapy, but recurrences are frequent (102). This infection can be life-threatening as it can be complicated by a liver abscess (rarely), septic thrombophlebitis or severe septicemia with visceral failure.

Recurrent acute cholangitis in patients with CDBD type IVA and type V is thought to be due to persistent bacterial colonization of the intrahepatic dilatations and to the possible presence of stones.

It is possible to manage an acute cholangitis episode by medical treatment (mainly antibiotic therapy) but recurrences favored by biliary stasis in the cyst seems inevitable in the absence of surgical management of the CDBD (103).

1.2. Acute Cholecystitis

This is a rare complication, but it may reveal the CDBD (104).

2. Mechanical Complications

According to the study by Urushihara N et al. (25) on PBMJ, there are some statistically significant associations as following:

- PBMJ Type A (Japanese classification) is associated with a younger age of patients and a higher rate of CDBD.
- The non-dilated CBD is more frequent with PBMJ type B.
- PBMJ Types B and C are associated with abdominal pain and high levels of amylasemia.
- PBMJ Type C is associated with more protein plugging (at the main pancreatic ductal level) and more biliary perforation.

2.1. Biliary Lithiasis

The reported frequency of intra cystic lithiasis ranges from 25 to 38% of cases. Biliary stasis favors the constitution of concretions leading to gallstone formation. These concretions can also develop in the residual intra-pancreatic part of the choledochal cyst, if the removal of the cyst has left an "eggcup bottom".

The simple common channel laying out with a moderate and diffuse dilatation of the entire extra hepatic bile ducts, favors oftenly the formation of a lithiasis of the lower part of the CBD (1, 105).

In the case of PBMJ, the CBD and gallbladder lithiasis occur more frequently in adults (23%) than in children (9%) (94).

2.2. Rupture of Choledochal Cyst

Spontaneous rupture is rare with an incidence ranging between 1.8 and 2%. In the majority of cases, it occurs in children under 4 years old.

The usual site of the rupture is the junction of the cystic duct with the common hepatic duct (50%). It can also occur in the distal part of the cyst (25%), or at the junction of the cyst with the left hepatic duct (106).

The cause of this complication is not clear yet. Pregnancy has been reported as a possible risk factor of spontaneous rupture of a bile duct cyst (107).

There are 3 modes of cyst rupture (91):

- A complete rupture with biliary peritonitis.
- A stuffy perforation of a bile duct cyst.
- Intramural perforation of the bile duct cyst. It remains covered by the serosa of the cyst.

The clinical presentation is usually a progressive abdominal distension, vomiting and possibly a septic shock with or without jaundice (1).

PBMJ Type C (according to the Japanese classification) and the fusiform type of CDBD (Todani type Ic) are significantly associated with frequent cystic perforation (107).

Traumatic rupture is rarer: only a few cases have been published.

2.3. Compression of Neighboring Structures

The cyst can push out neighboring organs with or without functional repercussions.

For example, a giant cyst can cause (48):

- Compression of the right ureter with right hydronephrosis, or
- Compression of the portal vein with portal hypertension as a consequence.

2.4. Acute Pancreatitis

It has been reported that the frequency of acute pancreatitis associated with CDBD is 10.5-56% in adults.

Transient abdominal pain due to protein plugs and hyperamylasemia are characteristic. However, these may also be misdiagnosed as acute pancreatitis (104).

3. Secondary Biliary Cirrhosis

Repeated obstruction and infections of CDBD (especially in patients with intrahepatic bile ducts dilatation), lead to the late occurrence of secondary biliary cirrhosis in 40-50% of patients. In this case, patients may also present with symptoms of portal hypertension such as gastrointestinal bleeding, splenomegaly and pancytopenia (103).

4. Malignant Degeneration

The complication that physicians fear most is the development of a malignant tumor of the bile ducts. Patients with CDBD would have a 6-30% risk of developing cholangiocarcinoma, which is much higher than the low prevalence of usual cholangiocarcinoma. Indeed, the risk of degeneration would be 20 times higher in patients with CDBD than in the general population (7).

A recent Japanese study reported a prevalence of 35% of cholangiocarcinoma in patients with CDBD associated with PBMJ. The latter is considered to be a risk factor for biliary carcinogenesis.

In addition, significant concentrations of carcinogenic substances have been noticed in the bile contents in case of PBMJ. However, the cause-effect relationship between PBMJ and cholangiocarcinoma has not been demonstrated yet.

According to Benavide MG et al. (108), patients with PBMJ and CDBD have a 21% risk of cholangiocarcinoma (62% as gallbladder cancer and 32% as CBD cancer), whereas patients presenting PBMJ without CDBD have a higher risk of cholangiocarcinoma at 42% (88% for gallbladder site and 7% for CBD location). It is worth noting that these tumors occur 15 to 20 years earlier than the general population.

The carcinogenesis mode of this type of cholangiocarcinoma associated with CDBD and/or PBMJ is the "hyperplasia-dysplasia-carcinoma" model, unlike the classic cholangiocarcinoma which arise according to the "adenoma-adenocarcinoma" sequence.

It should be noted that in case of PBMJ, the calculo-cancer of the gallbladder is very rare (64).

The percentage of degeneration is proportional to the age at which the CDBD is discovered: it reaches 0.7% in patients under 10 years old, 6.8% in patients between 11 and 20 years old, and 50% when the cyst is discovered after the age of 50 (109).

All types of CDBD are affected by the risk cancer, but the highest risk is associated with CDBD types I and IV of Todani classification. This risk is lower in type V, and it is lowest in CDBD types II and III.

Advanced age, cystic duct stenosis and incomplete choledochal cyst resection are associated with a high risk of cholangiocarcinoma (110-112).

The radiological diagnosis of CDBD degeneration is based mainly on the finding of localized or diffuse thickening of the cystic wall. In addition, the radiologist should search carefully for a suspicious thickening of the wall because it conditions both the therapeutic management and the prognosis.

Figure 10-1 shows an example of cholangiocarcinoma arising in a CDBD Todani type IVa.

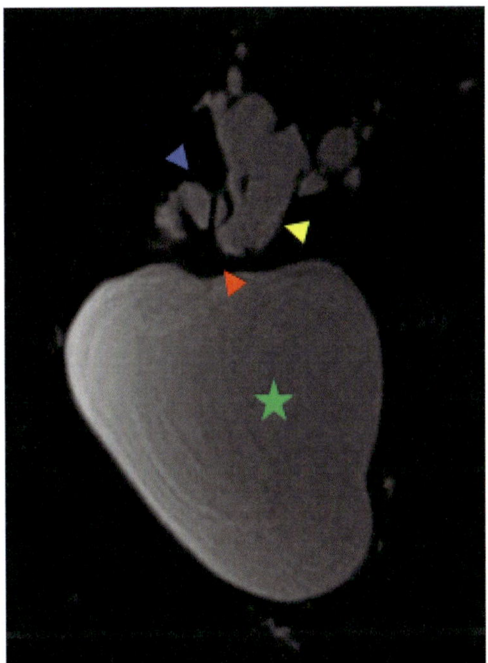

Figure 10-1: MRCP showing an area of bile duct thickening (red arrow head) between the choledochal cyst (green stars), the common hepatic duct (yellow arrow head) and cystic duct insertion (blue arrow head).

CHAPTER 11

TREATMENT OF CDBD

1. The Treatment Objectives

The treatment of CDBD is exclusively surgical: its main objectives are:

- To restore the normal flow of bile to the digestive tract,
- To suppress the reflux of pancreatic juice,
- To prevent or treat a complication, and
- To reduce the risk of degeneration (108).

Abstention (non-treatment option) leads to 97% mortality (34).

2. Therapeutic Methods

2.1. Medical Treatment

This is a necessary preoperative step, especially in case of complications such as acute cholangitis.

2.1.1. Correction of metabolic disorders

During septicemia with or without renal insufficiency, the correction of metabolic disturbances is essential by means of intravenous infusion to re-establish hydro-electrolytic and nutritional balance, to correct hypovolemia (by vascular filling under control of central venous pressure and diuresis), to fight against metabolic acidosis and to ensure an adequate supply of vitamin K if the prothrombin level is low.

2.1.2. Antibiotherapy in case of bile infection

Its aim is to control local infection and hematogenous bacterial spread by sterilizing tissue lesions. Associated cholestasis does not prevent normal or high liver tissue concentration of antibiotics, while it reduces their excretion in the bile.

It is generally a broad-spectrum probabilistic antibiotic therapy targeting Gram-negative bacilli and anaerobes: it combines Aminoside, Ampicillin and Metronidazole.

2.2. Endoscopic Treatment

Endoscopic sphincterotomy can be a temporary solution in case of acute cholangitis because it ensures free flow of bile and allows spontaneous or instrumental evacuation of gallstones. However, it can be difficult to perform in cases of PBMJ.

Endoscopic treatment can in no case substitute curative surgical treatment of CDBD (110).

2.3. Interventional Radiology

Percutaneous biliary drainage consists of puncturing the bile ducts by trans-hepatic route under ultrasound and/or CT scan control with drain installation. Its success rate is close to 100% when the bile ducts are dilated. The puncture is done with a fine needle, usually on the right bile ducts by a right intercostal approach, or more rarely by a trans-epigastrium path.

There are three types of percutaneous drainage (113):

- *External drainage:* where the catheter is placed upstream of the obstacle. It allows the bile to be drained to the outside. The indication of this type of drainage is an emergency context with acute cholangitis to limit handling and drain outside the infected bile.
- *Internal-external drainage:* where the catheter is placed through stenosis (the area of obstruction), communicating the bile ducts downstream of the obstacle with the bile ducts upstream of it and with the external environment.
- *Internal drainage or endoprosthesis:* consists of placing a metal stent or a plastic prosthesis at the obstruction site to ensure that the canal is open and the bile flows out.

2.4. Surgical Treatment

2.4.1. Surgery approaches

Open surgery for CDBD resection with entero-biliary reconstruction is the standard procedure performed by midline laparotomy or at best by right sub-costal laparotomy.

For some teams the exclusive *laparoscopic approach* is possible especially for children. Zheng J et al. (114) recently published (in 2020) a study of 325 children operated on for CDBD under laparoscopy, comparing subjects less than 3 months old (19 patients) with the other 306 children aged between 3 months and 6 years. The overall conversion rate was 1.2% and the overall post-operative complication rate was 7.1%. However, this study showed that the group of infants under 3 months old had a significantly higher operative duration, length of hospital stay, conversion rate and early post-operative morbidity rate.

A Turkish study (115), also published in 2020, involved 8 adult patients operated on by laparoscopy for CDBD type I (7 cases) or IV (1 case) of Todani classification. The median operating time was 330 minutes (240 - 480 minutes) and only one patient had a conversion to laparotomy. There were 3 cases of biliary fistula managed non-operatively. This shows that a lot of expertise is required for laparoscopic treatment of DKVB.

The robotic approach has been shown to be feasible and satisfactory in children with results broadly comparable to laparoscopy ones and even open surgery outcomes (116).

The Chinese study of Chi S et al. (117), recently published in 2020, retrospectively compared the 2 laparoscopic and robotic approaches in 140 patients (70 in each group) who underwent CDBD excision (Todani type I or IV) with entero-biliary anastomosis. From a technical point of view, laparoscopy had a significantly lower operating time, but robotic surgery had not only significantly higher exposure rates of the right and left hepatic ducts and the intra-pancreatic portion of the common bile duct, but also a significantly shorter operating time of performing an entero-biliary anastomosis. In addition, in terms of the overall rate of early post-operative complications, robotic surgery was significantly better.

2.4.2. Surgical methods

2.4.2.1. The old methods

- *External drainage:* after choledochotomy and t-tube (Kehr drain) installation. This option can be considered in cases of acute cholangitis, cyst perforation, cyst fissuration, and acute pancreatitis.
- *Internal drainage:* this may be done as a cysto-duodenostomy or a cysto-jejunostomy with an excluded jejunal loop (Roux-en-Y) which is more effective in preventing intra-biliary reflux. This seems to be a simple solution but physician should not opt for it for several reasons: the high rate of symptoms recurrence, the high rate of re-interventions and the high risk of secondary cholangiocarcinoma.

Indeed, the overall success rate of internal drainage is 30%, while the risk of postoperative malignancy is 30%, the mortality rate is 11% and more than half of the patients will require re-intervention (118).

- *Hepaticojejunostomy with CDBD exclusion:* this technique was described by HEPP. The first of this intervention consists of sectioning the hepatic duct upstream of the cyst if it is of a suitable size (wide enough, not too narrow), otherwise the surgeon should preserve a collarette of the upper pole of the cyst for a quite wide entero-biliary anastomosis. The choledochal cyst is then closed without any resection. A hepaticojejunostomy is then performed with a Roux-en-Y excluded jejunal loop. The main risk of this method is pancreatic reflux into the cystic cavity, particularly due to an underlying PBMJ. However, there is a major risk of malignant transformation of the non-resected choledochal cyst. At present, this treatment of CDBD is considered not only incomplete, but above all dangerous (119).

2.4.2.2. The reference methods

- *Total resection of the choledochal cyst with bilio-enteric anastomosis:* it was first proposed by Mac Werther in 1924. Total resection of the cyst followed by hepaticojejunostomy with a Roux-en-Y jejunal loop is currently the treatment of choice as it ensures biliary derivation and reduces the risk of neoplastic degeneration to less than 1%. From a technical point of view, this resection must be as total as possible and go upwards on the common hepatic duct, or even at the level of biliary convergence, based on radiological and per operative findings. Towards the bottom, pancreatic parenchyma and Wirsung injuries must be avoided and the ligation of the distal common bile duct must be done just upstream of the second portion of the duodenum (120).
- *Duodeno-pancreatectomy:* is a disproportionate gesture. Nevertheless, it should be performed in case of degeneration of either the intra pancreatic bile duct or the long common duct (of a PBMJ) but so far, no case has been reported in the literature.
- *Surgical exploration before CDBD surgery:*
  - Intra-operative cholangiography allows the determination of the CDBD anatomical type (according to Todani classification) and the search for a possible PBMJ.

- The liver may be normal, retentional or cirrhotic in appearance. Thus, a liver biopsy is suitable to look for histological signs of hepatic fibrosis or cirrhosis.
- The condition of the pancreas must also be assessed because of possible chronic pancreatitis.
- An extemporaneous pathological examination of the resected CDBD limit is only recommended if a cholangiocarcinoma is suspected.

▪ *Methods of choledochal cyst excision:*
  - **Total resection:** the simplest and most careful method is to section the cyst at its middle part and then to dissect its upper pole from bottom to top: the surgeon should preserve the biliary convergence (if possible: this means that there is no intra-hepatic bile ducts cystic dilation) for a simple and easier entero-biliary anastomosis. Subsequently, dissection of the lower pole is carried out gradually. The total resection should be easy and simple if the cystic pouch ends at the upper edge of the pancreas. In this situation, the normal distal part of the common bile duct, is simply sutured with an absorbable thread (120).
  - **Partial resection:** if the choledochal cyst is in close contact with the head of the pancreas, the risk of the Wirsung duct injury is then high. This may justify a partial resection of the cyst (121). In this case, the lower end of the dilated part of the bile duct is left in situ as an "eggcup bottom".

▪ *Segmental, lobar or atypical hepatic resections:* these options are indicated in case of intrahepatic degeneration or a one-sided intra hepatic bile duct dilatation (Todani type IVa or V).

▪ *Liver transplantation:* it is recommended in case of secondary biliary cirrhosis or an extensive Caroli's disease.

3. Treatment Indications

3.1. Indications for Surgical Treatment

Entero-cystic diversions should be prohibited.

The surgical approach differs according to the type of CDBD. However, it must take into consideration certain criteria: the age of the patient, his general condition, the possible complication and the preoperative imaging and the intraoperative cholangiography findings.

3.1.1. CDBD type I

Surgical resection should involve the gallbladder and the entire CBD. It should also preserve the roof of the biliary convergence on the top and a millimeter-sized portion of the intra-pancreatic portion of the choledocus at the bottom (121). Complications such as hemorrhage, acute pancreatitis, biliary fistula, pancreatic fistula and even papillary disinsertion can occur especially in the case of extensive and traumatic dissection of the intra-pancreatic bile duct.

Cephalic duodeno-pancreatectomy should be prohibited in the absence of cholangiocarcinoma.

3.1.2. CDBD type II

It is commonly admitted that excision of the cyst (biliary diverticulum) alone is adequate. However, cholecystectomy is also recommended if there is a PBMJ BPA because of the high risk of gallbladder malignancy even in the absence gallbladder stones.

The surgery of type II CDBD has usually a low risk of complications.

When the cyst is densely adherent to the underlying portal vein, it is suitable to use Lilly's technique which consists in taking away the mucosal layer while a part of the adventitia of the cyst wall is left against the portal vein. This is the internal "peeling" method (53, 122).

In most cases, the method of choice is the same as that used for CDBD type I. Indeed, this ensures an excision of the entire diverticulum and cholecystectomy but a hepatico-jejunal anastomosis must be performed (114).

3.1.3. CDBD type III

CDBD type III has a very low risk of malignant transformation (123). Therefore, excision of the cyst with the whole extra hepatic bile ducts is considered too radical.

Endoscopic sphincterotomy or cystostomy is currently considered the treatment of choice for these patients.

In the case of symptomatic choledocele, the physician may opt for a simple incision of the cyst (cystostomy) or for partial cyst excision with being careful not to damage biliary and pancreatic ducts implantations (124). The main goal of these options (particularly mini-invasive endoscopic cystotomy) is to avoid intra cystic bile retention.

3.1.4. CDBD type IV

The complete surgical excision of the extra-hepatic biliary tree is mandatory for CDBD type IVB and for the extra-hepatic part of CDBD type IVA (96).

However, the management of the intra-hepatic part of CDBD type IVA is far from being consensual and several authors suggest different approaches as following:

- Lipsett and Pitt (125) propose a non-resection attitude with insertion of a trans hepatic stent so as to facilitate post operative extraction of possible calculi.
- However, many other authors are in favor of liver resection, as it completely eradicates both the extra-hepatic and intra-hepatic components of the disease. This is clearly recommended in case of intra-hepatic bile ducts cystic dilation limited to the left liver lobe.
- Considering patients with CDBD type IVA and bi-lobal dilatation of intra hepatic bile ducts, several studies found that a large proportions of them showed regression or even disappearance of intra hepatic bile ducts dilatation after CBD resection and Roux-en-Y termino lateral hepaticojejunostomy (126).
- Hemonta KD et al. (127) suggest to perform a mucosectomy on the biliary stump (or residual cystic bile duct) to be used for hepaticojejunostomy after CBD resection possibly with unilobar hepatectomy. The benefit of this technique would be to avoid or reduce as much as possible the risk of hepaticojejunostomy complications, namely stenosis, cholangitis, intrahepatic lithiasis and cholangiocarcinoma. This technique could be a good alternative in case of bi-lobal intrahepatic dilatation.

According to the same author, mucosectomy is usually technically easy because the cleavage plane between the pathological mucosa and the rest of the wall is relatively easy to find.

3.1.5. CDBD Todani type V

The CDBD Type V cyst (Caroli disease) is a rare type that is not always easy to manage.

The choice of treatment strategy must take into account two important factors:

- First, the extent of the intra-hepatic disease (uni- or bilobar) and
- second, the presence of an associated chronic hepatic pathology (hepatic fibrosis, secondary biliary cirrhosis and cholangiocarcinoma) (96):
  - For unilobar intrahepatic disease with normal hepatic parenchyma, liver resection seems to be the best treatment with good long-term outcomes (128).
  - Conservative surgery (without any hepatic resection) is associated with a high risk of recurrent episodes of cholangitis and upper gastrointestinal hemorrhage (due to ruptured varicose veins) either in the context of coexisting pathologic hepatic parenchyma (congenital liver fibrosis or secondary biliary cirrhosis) with or without portal hypertension, or in case of bilobar intra hepatic ducts cystic dilation. Therefore, liver transplantation is considered the treatment of choice in these situations (48, 129).

3.1.6. CDBD (new) type VI

The treatment of a this CDBD type VI depends closely on the connection between the cystic duct (of the gallbladder) and the CBD (3). Two situations are possible:

- *Situation 1:* there is a fine and usual communication between the cystic duct (or cyst) and the common bile duct which is not dilated. This is an indication for a cholecystectomy removing the cystic duct and the cyst. It can be performed either laparoscopically or under open surgery.
- *Situation 2:* there is a wide communication between the cystic duct (or cyst) and the common bile duct. In this case, the latter is oftenly wide or dilated. This is an indication for cholecystectomy and total resection of the CBD with termino lateral hepaticojejunostomy.

It is worth noting that chemotherapy, based on Cisplatin-Gemcitabine, is highly recommended in case of vesicular tumors associated to CDBD type VI and with the following characteristics: T2, N+ or residual tumor (130).

3.1.7. PBMJ

Patients with PBMJ should undergo preventive cholecystectomy even in the absence of bile duct dilatation and gallbladder stones (22, 23).

The Japanese guidelines (63, 131) of 2012 for the therapeutic strategy of a PBMJ are as follows:

- PBMJ with CDBD: cholecystectomy with CDBD resection and hepaticojejunostomy.
- PBMJ without CDBD: prophylactic cholecystectomy, even for completely asymptomatic patients, due to a high risk of gallbladder cancer. Furthermore, there is not enough evidence to recommend a systematic resection of the CBD.

It is worth noting that in the case of PBMJ, the association of vesicular lithiasis and gallbladder cancer is very rare (64).

3.1.8. Enterobiliary anastomosis after choledochal cyst resection

Several publications, mainly concerning pediatric cases (Table 11-1), including a meta-analysis (132) published in 2013, have compared the results of termino lateral hepaticoduodenostomy and hepaticojejunostomy after CDBD resection. These studies showed the feasibility of hepaticoduodenostomy in this context and even its superiority in terms of operating time and hospital stay. This is illustrated in tables 11-1 and 11-2. However, the hepaticoduodenostomy is clearly associated to a high risk of gastroduodenal reflux with gastritis and epigastric pain. This would require in the most of cases to transform the hepaticoduodenostomy into a hepaticojejunostomy if a treatment with proton pump inhibitor is not enough.

Table 11-1: Results of studies comparing HDS and AHJ

Study	Year	Surgical approach	Number of patients	Age of patients	Results
Sarath KN (132) ***Meta-analysis***	2013	Laparoscopy 1 study: 99%. 5 studies: 15%.	679 HDS: 412 HJS: 267	5 studies: < 10 years 1 study: 27 days - 25 years	- H Stay: HDS << HJS - R/G: HDS >>> HJS - OT, BF, AC, AS, RI: HDS ≈ HJS
Fanny Y (49) ***Retrospective study***	2015	Laparoscopy	54 patients HDS: 21 HJS: 33	10 - 83 months (< 7 years old)	- H Stay and OT: HDS << HJS - R/G, BF, AC, AS, RI: HDS ≈ HJS

AC: acute cholangitis; AS: anastomotic stenosis; BF: biliary fistula; H: hospital; OT: Operative time; PPI: proton pump inhibitors; R/G: reflux/gastritis; RI: re-intervention; >>> or <<: significant difference; ≈: non-significant difference

Table 11-2: Results of studies about HDS

Study	Year	Surgical approach	Number of patients	Age of patients	Results
Patil V (133) ***Retrospective study***	2012	Right subcostal laparotomy	54 patients - 40 < 12 YO - 14 > 12 YO	Mean: 18 YO (3 M – 36 YO)	- BF without return: 2 cases - AS: 1 case after 18 years
Hamada Y (134) ***Retrospective study***	2017	Unspecified	17	Mean: 4.2 YO (11 days - 18 YO)	With a FU of 17 years (14 - 22) - R/G: 100% after 5.4 years - AC, AS, APD: 14 patients, 9 of whom had RI with HDS converted to HJS - After 12.6 years (8-16 years) No recidivism after RI
Nazki S (116) ***Retrospective study***	2020	Robotics	19	Mean: 7 YO (2.5 – 14 YO)	- Mean OT: 170 ± 40 minutes After a FU of 2.5 years (0.5 - 3.5 years) - Minimal APD: 5 patients - R/G: 1 patient treated with PPI - RI: none

AC: acute cholangitis; AS: anastomotic stenosis; APD: abdominal pain and discomfort; BF: biliary fistula; FU: Follow-Up; OT: Operative time; PPI: proton pump inhibitors; R/G: reflux/gastritis; RI: re-intervention; YO: years-old

3.2. Indications for Endoscopic Treatment

Endoscopic sphincterotomy is indicated for small choledoceles. It is also indicated in case of CDBD with a CBD lithiasis causing a severe cholangitis.

This therapeutic option remains a temporary solution for fragile patients at high surgical risk.

3.3. Special Cases

Even though the intervention principle remains the same with total resection of the common bile duct and bilio-digestive anastomosis; certain circumstances due to anatomical variations or to a complication can make pre and per operative exploration and surgery more difficult.

3.3.1. In an infectious context

Bile retention is the main cause of the cyst infection. So, it is urgent to ensure biliary drainage. This complication is usually diagnosed during a first outbreak of acute cholangitis. However, it happens that cyst infection is discovered during surgery.

In the case of severe infection, percutaneous and trans-hepatic drainage of the bile duct should be considered as a first step, while ensuring that there is no perforation or intra-peritoneal bile leakage. Then, a radical intervention (surgery) should be done as soon as possible.

It is worth noting that surgery is generally more difficult in case of local inflammatory changes (caused by a recent infection) or if the patient has a history of previous abdominal operation (135).

3.3.2. CDBD and CBD lithiasis

In some cases where the dilatation upstream of the calculus is only fusiform and non-cystic in nature, the question may even arise as to the possible role of this lithiasis in the bile ducts dilatation. However, it does not seem reasonable to remove CBD lithiasis without any biliary resection, when it is associated to a PBMJ.

In adults, it may be sometimes preferable to opt first for endoscopic sphincterotomy before surgery particularly if there is a stone in the common channel of a PBMJ.

3.3.3. CDBD and cirrhosis

The CDBD may cause early and severe hepatic parenchymal repercussion as the development of cirrhosis, especially in the youngest children. This may lead to portal hypertension. Thus, surgical dissection would be much more difficult and hemorrhagic.

It is worth noting that cirrhosis and portal hypertension can mask the CDBD and thus delay its diagnosis in adulthood.

3.3.4. Cholangiocarcinoma arising in CDBD

It is the main feared complication of CDBD. Cholangiocarcinoma develops either on extra hepatic bile ducts, particularly if there has never been any previous biliary intervention, or on intra hepatic bile ducts, especially if it remained very dilated after CBD resection.

The preoperative diagnosis of degeneration in CDBD is not always easy, and cholangiocarcinoma may be made discovered during surgery or by an extemporaneous histological examination.

Generally, the hepatic and lymph node extension is too important that any lymph node dissection illusory and the prognosis of such cholangiocarcinoma (due to CDBD) remain very poor (136).

Indeed, this cholangiocarcinoma is oftenly diagnosed at an advanced stage with biliary retention and wide extension. Thus, frequently, the only therapeutic possibility is an internal bypass (or a biliary prothesis) of a palliative nature (136).

3.3.5. CDBD with gallbladder agenesis

In the case of gallbladder agenesis, biliary ducts dilation could be explained by biliary stasis and thus CDBD may be misdiagnosed.

The presence of chronic dilatation of the CBD with gallbladder agenesis should be led to a CBD resection with termino-lateral hepaticojejunostomy so as to avoid the risk of secondary cholangiocarcinoma (137).

CHAPTER 12

PROGNOSIS

1. Mortality

The prognosis of CDBD has been steadily improving over the years, thanks to: the high performance of new imaging modalities (allowing precise and early diagnosis), better scientific knowledge concerning CDBD as well as to the surgical techniques' improvement. Indeed, in 1935 the mortality rate was 90% whereas currently it is 5%.

Even though, the mortality rate for all possible surgical procedures for CDBD has considerably decreased, the method of choice remains scystic biliary ducts resection with a termino-lateral Roux-en-Y hepaticojejunostomy (49).

The age of patient at the moment of CDBD diagnosis is a major prognosis factor. In fact, the prognosis is poor for infants with CDBD and the risk of biliary cirrhosis remains very high even after an adequate surgery.

2. Morbidity

Numerous postoperative complications have been reported:

2.1. Early complications

- *Infectious complications:*
  They are mainly:
  - Abdominal wall infection.
  - Subhepatic abscess: this means that the physician should look for an anastomotic biliary leakage.
  - Acute cholangitis.
  - Septicemia.
- *Biliary complications* (96):
  - External biliary fistula.
  - A localized collection biliary or biloma.
  - Choleperitoneum or biliary peritonitis.

- *Liver failure:*

  It is mainly seen in children in cases of biliary cirrhosis and possibly after liver excision.

2.2. Late complications

- *Stenosis or obliteration of the bilio-enteric anastomosis:*

  It can be responsible for recurrent jaundice, abdominal pain or acute cholangitis. This complication usually requires a re-intervention.

  Jung K et al. showed in their study that CDBD Todani type IA is more likely to cause (bilio-enteric) anastomotic stenosis than Todani types IC and IVA (96). However, the study of Kim JH (139) found that CDBD Todani type IVA is significantly associated with more hepaticojejunostomy stenosis than type IA.

  According to the same study (139), there is 3 risk factors of hepaticojejunostomy stenosis, done in the context of CDBD. They are as following:

  - Elderly patient.
  - The size of the cyst: the average size of the choledochal cyst associated with postoperative hepaticojejunostomy stenosis is 7 cm whereas the average size of the choledochal cysts that didn't have this postoperative complication is 4cm.
  - The preoperative duration of symptoms: it is significantly shorter in the hepaticojejunostomy stenosis group (compared averages: 27 days Versus 483 days).

  In addition, this study (139) showed also that there is a correlation between the inflammation degree of the CDBD wall and 3 parameters, namely the size of the cyst, the thickness of the pathological biliary wall and the loss of biliary mucosa.

- *Intra-cystic and gallbladder lithiasis:*

  The risk of developing biliary lithiasis after surgery for CDBD is approximatively 10% (57).

  This complication seems to be frequent in case of persistent cystic pouch. Its main symptom is the comeback of abdominal pain which is frequently associated with fluctuating jaundice. This will inevitably lead to a reoperation.

  The pigmentary type is the most common type of this kind of lithiasis (57).

- *Secondary cholangitis:*

  This is a relatively frequent complication if there is a persistent dilation of the intra-hepatic bile ducts, even discreetly. Furthermore, this secondary cholangitis is a real risk factor of malignant degeneration.

  The patients who underwent surgery for CDBD Todani type IVA and those who have recurrent post operative acute cholangitis must be closely monitored for life because of high risk of biliary cholangiocarcinoma (139).

- *Cholangiocarcinoma:*

  Generally, this complication occurs in case of persistent (even discrete) dilation of intra-hepatic bile ducts after CBD resection. This is why several authors recommended that these patients should have a close follow-up after surgery, for a minimum of 10 years (123) or at best for life (64, 140).

  The risk of cholangiocarcinoma in patients within CDBD associated with PBMJ, is clearly greater in non-operated patients than in patients who have had a bilio-digestive bypass (131).

  Squamous cell carcinoma of the bile ducts is an extremely rare complication of CDBD. Surgery is the only curative therapeutic option. Nevertheless, its prognosis still very poor. Moreover, adjuvant radiation therapy and chemotherapy is useless and derisory (141).

  Finally, it is worth noting that there is a very minimal risk of pancreatic cancer in patients with PBMJ after surgery (142).

CHAPTER 13

CONCLUSION

CDBD is a congenital biliary malformation that presents as an abnormal dilatation of part or all of the bile ducts without any lithiasis or tumor obstruction. This abnormality must be obvious on imaging. It is generally associated with a PBMJ.

CDBD is the most common congenital condition of the biliary tree after bile ducts atresia. It affects the female sex more frequently. It can be diagnosed in childhood. However, it can remain asymptomatic for a long time and the diagnosis is only made at adulthood or even at an advanced age.

The advent of Bili-IRM has revolutionized the diagnosis of CDBD. In addition, the CPRM is currently crucial for the choice of therapeutic strategy

In 1977, Todani and his colleagues developed the most widely used CDBD classification. This is a classification into 5 types of which type I is the most common (80%).

Nevertheless, several recent publications suggest a new type of CDBD affecting the cystic duct (of the gallbladder) alone or in association with another type of the CDBD Todani classification. Indeed, isolated dilatation of the cystic duct does not belong to any of the 5 types of the Todani classification. This is why many authors think that this anomaly should be classified as Todani type VI or as a subgroup of Todani type II.

At present, it is well established that CDBD is the consequence of a PBMJ according to Babbit's theory. However, this theory does not explain CDBD in the absence of any PBMJ. This is why other etiologies have been suggested such as viral cause and the bile ducts denervation. In addition, there is an embryological hypothesis which states that PBMJ is linked to malrotation of the pancreatic ventral bud. In this case, the fusion of the two ventral and dorsal pancreatic buds could take place in an oblique position which leads to the formation of a long common duct.

The old definition of the PBMJ is based on several pathological criteria:

- one major criterion, namely the presence of a common biliopancreatic channel known as the "long common channel" with a minimal length of 10mm in adults,

- and two minor criteria: the first is an extra duodenal bilio-pancreatic junction upstream of the Oddi sphincter. The second is a bilio-pancreatic connection angle of more than 30°.

According to the new Japanese recommendations of the JSPBM ("Japanese Study Group of Pancreato-biliary Maljunction") published in 2015, the PBMJ is currently defined as a biliopancreatic junction located outside the duodenal wall, revealed by imaging and possibly confirmed by histological examination. According to this scholarly society, 2 other secondary but not necessary criteria may help diagnosing PBMJ: these are the presence of a CDBD and high level of biliary amylases.

PBMJ were previously classified by Kimura (simple classification into 2 types) and by Komi (more elaborate classification into 3 types). However, the JSPBM classifies PBMJ into 4 types A, B, C and D.

CDBD is mainly diagnosed in childhood (75%) with typical symptoms whereas it presents atypically in adults because the symptoms become less discernible. Indeed, the most classic mode of CDBD discovery involves Bernheim's clinical triad with a palpable mass of the right hypochondrium, jaundice and right hypochondrium pain. However, this triad would only be present in 6 to 20% of cases, whereas patients usually present with one or two symptoms of this triad.

Furthermore, CDBD may be asymptomatic or rarely discovered during complications such as biliary perforation, biliary and hepatic infection, acute pancreatitis, biliary lithiasis, cirrhosis with portal hypertension and malignant degeneration.

The presence of PBMJ with CDBD is associated with a 21% risk of cholangiocarcinoma (62% for gallbladder cancer and 32% for CBD cancer) whereas PBMJ without CDBD is associated with a higher risk (42%) of secondary cholangiocarcinoma (88% in the gallbladder site and 7% in the CBD). It is worth noting that this kind of tumor occurs 15 to 20 years earlier than the general population.

This type of cholangiocarcinoma secondary to CDBD and PBMJ occurs in the "hyperplasia-dysplasia-carcinoma" mode, unlike the classic cholangiocarcinoma which follows the "adenoma-adenocarcinoma" sequence.

All types of CDBD are concerned with malignant transformation. However, the highest risk was found with CDBD Todani types I and IV. This risk is lower in type V, and it is lowest in types II and III.

The Bili-IRM (CPRM) is the reference imaging modality for a thorough exploration of the biliary and pancreatic ducts. This examination is very sensitive (70% to 100%) and highly specific (90% to 100%) in the diagnosis and classification of CDBD. It also allows a reliable identification of a PBMJ (in particular with secretin injection) as well as of possible cholangiocarcinoma and biliary (CBD) lithiasis.

From a therapeutic standpoint, cysto-digestive derivations should be avoided.

The surgical strategy differs according to the type of malformation as following:

- For type I: The surgical resection must involve the gallbladder and the entire CBD and have to preserve the roof of the biliary convergence at the top and a millimeter-sized portion of the intra-pancreatic choledocus at the bottom.
- For type II or biliary diverticulum. As there is a very a low risk of complications, it is commonly accepted that excision of the cyst (or diverticulum) alone is adequate.
- For Type III: endoscopic sphincterotomy is currently considered the reference treatment.
- For type IV: the complete surgical excision of the extra-hepatic biliary tree is recommended for the CDBD type IVB and for the extra-hepatic component of CDBD type IVA. However, the management of the intra-hepatic component of CDBD type IVA is far from being consensual. Indeed, some authors propose a conservative attitude because they noticed many cases with intra hepatic bile ducts dilatation vanishing after this type of surgery). A second group of authors recommend a left or right hepatectomy depending on the most affected side by CDBD. In addition, other authors recommend performing a mucosectomy on the biliary stump (or residual cystic bile duct) because it would avoid or reduce as much as possible the risk of hepaticojejunostomy complications namely stenosis, acute cholangitis, intrahepatic lithiasis and cholangiocarcinoma. This mucosectomy could be a good alternative in case of bi-lobal intrahepatic dilatation.
- For Type V: two treatment options are possible. First, patients with non-pathological hepatic parenchyma should undergo right or left liver resection for unilateral intrahepatic CDBD. Second, in case of congenital liver fibrosis or secondary biliary cirrhosis (with or without portal hypertension), or if both hepatic lobes are affected, liver transplantation is considered the treatment of choice.
- For type VI: A cholecystectomy with complete cystic duct (of the gallbladder) should be performed. In addition, a total resection of the CBD with termino-lateral Roux-en-Y hepaticojejunostomy is

recommended if there is wide communication between the cystic duct and the choledocus.
- In case of PBMJ without any associated CDBD: cholecystectomy is recommended because of the high risk of gallbladder cancer.
- The chronic dilation of the CBD in case of gallbladder agenesis should be an indication for CBD resection with hepaticojejunostomy because of the high risk of cholangiocarcinoma.
- Laparoscopy is a safe and effective approach, especially with experienced surgeons. Robotic surgery would also be as effective as laparoscopy.
- The only indication for cephalic duodeno-pancreatectomy is cholangiocarcinoma of the lower choledocus.

Anastomotic stenosis is one of the most frequent complications of hepaticojejunostomy performed after CDBD resection. The risk factors for this are advanced age, cyst size over 7 cm and short preoperative duration of the clinical symptoms.

Post-operative cholangiocarcinoma is usually seen in cases of persistent dilatation even discrete, of intra hepatic bile ducts. This is why patients should be monitored for a minimum period of 10 years and at best for life. Furthermore, patients operated for CDBD type IVA or with recurrent postoperative acute cholangitis must undergo a very long follow-up because of high risk of hepatic cirrhosis and mainly secondary cholangiocarcinoma.

PART 2

PANCREATIC DUCTS ANOMALIES

CHAPTER 1

INTRODUCTION

Congenital anomalies of the pancreas and pancreatic ducts are rare and usually asymptomatic. These anomalies are pancreas divisum, annular pancreas, Agenesis of the dorsal agenesis and ansa pancreatica. The most common of these malformations is the pancreas divisum.

These congenital anomalies are oftenly discovered fortuitously in patients explored for other causes. Their most common clinical presentation is recurrent acute pancreatitis and chronic pancreatitis.

The development of imaging techniques over the last few decades in particular the CPRM, raised the diagnosis rates of these malformations and allowed their better assessment. However, their management remains difficult and above all non-consensual to date.

In this chapter, we will review the epidemiological, physio pathological, clinical, morphological and therapeutic aspects of the different congenital pancreatic ductal anomalies.

CHAPTER 2

THE PANCREAS DIVISUM

Pancreas Divisum (PDiv) is the most common congenital pancreatic malformation. It results from a fusion flaw of the ductal systems of the dorsal and ventral pancreatic embryonic vestiges during the 7th week of embryonic life (1, 2). This leads to a canal configuration made up of a dominant dorsal pancreatic duct draining through the minor papilla, and a ventral pancreatic duct which drains through the major papilla (3,4).

1. Epidemiology

The prevalence of PDiv is between 6 and 10% of the general population according to autopsy series (3, 4), endoscopic studies (5, 6) and radiological explorations (7). The prevalence is slightly lower among Asians and Africans (6, 8).

There is no demonstrated masculine or feminine predominance.

The majority (95%) of symptom-free patients are accidentally discovered (9).

2. Embryology

During embryonic life, the pancreas appears at the level of the duodenal floor in the form of two rough outlines: the dorsal embryonic vestige and the ventral one. The latter, from which the hepatobiliary system will develop, joins the dorsal vestige under the effect of the anterior intestine rotation and the development of the hepatic outline.

The ventral vestige will form the major part of the pancreas head and the uncinus process. These pancreatic parts will develop below the dorsal outline.

The whole body and the tail of the pancreas derives from the dorsal vestige which will also contribute to the formation of a minor part of the pancreatic head.

The ventral and dorsal ductal systems merge at the level of the pancreatic isthmus. The segment of the dorsal duct located to the right of this fusion zone will constitute the corporeal-caudal part of the *main pancreatic duct* (the Wirsung duct). On the other hand, the left part of this duct (located to the left of this fusion zone) will become *the accessory pancreatic duct* (the Santorini duct) which drains into the duodenum at the level of the minor papilla.

The ventral pancreas duct will turn into the cephalic part of the main pancreatic duct which joins the bile duct (choledocus) to end in the major papilla known also as the Vater's ampulla (10, 11) (Figure 2-1).

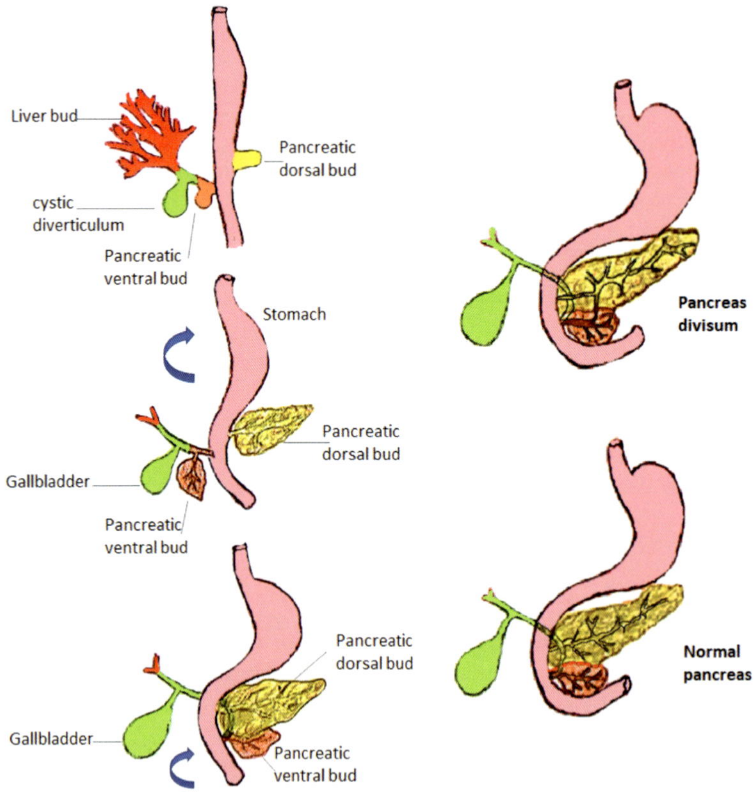

Figure 2-1: Pancreas divisum embrypgenesis: the 3 images at the left show the rotation of the pancreatic ventral bud to fuse with the dorsal pancreatic bud during the embryonic life. The pancreas divisum rsults from a fusion defect of the dorsal and the ventral ducts. This means that the major part of the pancreas drains into the dorsal pancreatic duct towards the minor papilla (image top right).

Taking into account the pancreas embryogenesis, the PDiv is clearly due to a fusion anomaly of the ventral and the dorsal ductal systems. It can be either a complete shortcoming fusion or a rudimentary fusion.

There is 3 main PDiv subtypes (Figure 2-2):

- *Complete PDiv:* this is the most typical and most frequent (70%) subtype of PDiv (1, 12). There is no communication between the dorsal and ventral ducts.
- *Incomplete PDiv:* its prevalence is 6-15% (13,14,15). In this case, the communication between the dorsal and ventral ducts is ensured by a fine, rudimentary branch which obviously poorly functioning. However, an opacification through the major papilla may show the dorsal duct.
- *Reverse PDiv:* this is a rare variant of PDiv. The accessory pancreatic duct known as the Santorini duct does not connect to the bend of the main pancreatic duct. This ductal interruption of the Santorini can sometimes be misinterpreted as a stenosis of benign or malignant origin. In addition, this entity may have no clinical expression.

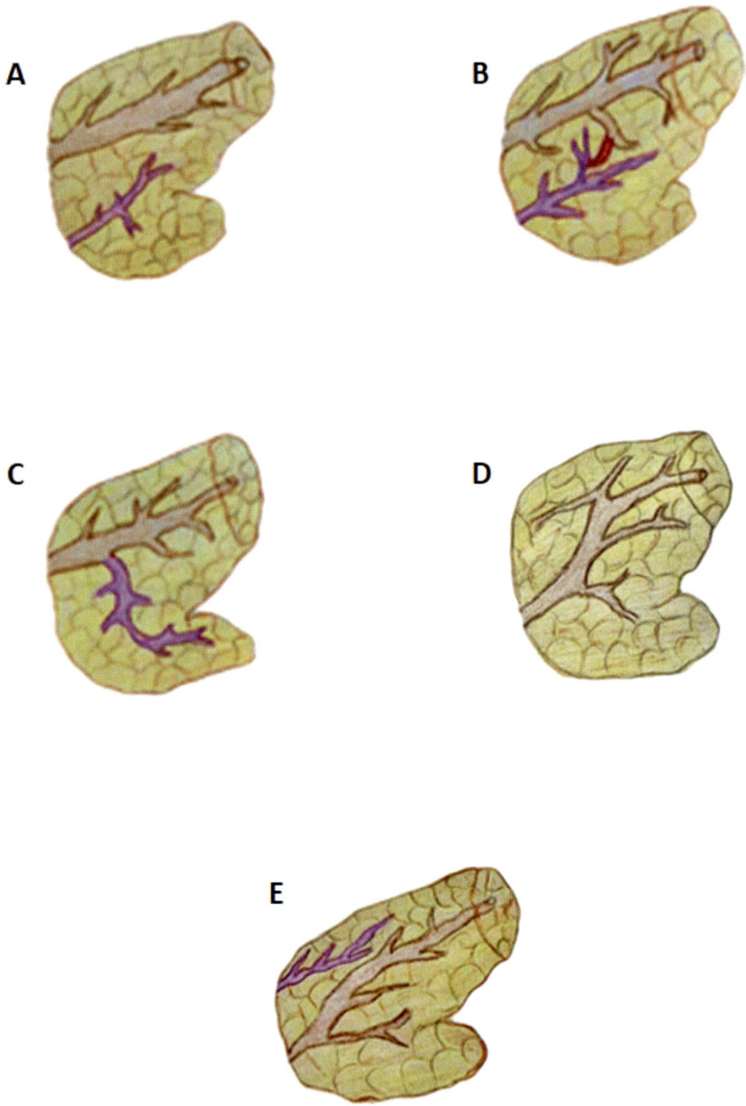

Figure 2-2: Types of pancreas divisum. A: type I or complete pancreas divisum (classic type); B: Type III or incomplete pancreas divisum; C: pancreas divisum with isolated dorsal duct; D: pancreas divisum with isolated ventral duct; E: inverted pancreas divisum. A, B and E are the 3 main types of pancreas divisum.

Three other PDiv subtypes have been also reported (Figure 2-2):

- *PDiv with an isolated ventral duct:* the accessory pancreatic channel does not end into the duodenum.
- *PDiv with an isolated dorsal duct:* the ventral pancreatic channel does not end into the duodenum or may even be absent. This subtype prevalence may reach 23% in certain series).
- *Pseudo PDiv / False PDiv:* An obstruction of the main pancreatic duct downstream the origin of the accessory Santorini duct (due to acute pancreatitis, a chronic pancreatitis ductal stenosis or a pancreatic tumor) can be mistaken for a complete pancreas divisum. This obstruction can lead to the atrophy of the head of the pancreas with a compensatory increase in the size of the accessory duct draining the body and the tail in this case. This gives an appearance mimicking that of the pancreas divisum on ERCP and CPRM images. Careful questioning of the patient and a thorough semiological analysis of these two types of imaging allows a correct diagnosis and specially to unmask a malignant lesion.

3. Associated Biliopancreatic Anomalies

PDiv can be associated with other pancreatic or biliary abnormalities in particular and mainly the Annular pancreas. Some studies have estimated the prevalence of this association at 30 to 38% (16-18) and a recent study has estimated that the association is of the order of 50% (19).

The other possible associated malformations reported in the literature are cystic dilation of bile ducts cystic, pancreato biliary maljunction (20-25) and partial agenesis of the dorsal pancreas. Some publications reported the association of the latter malformation with PDiv, but there is still debate as to the causality of the two conditions in relation to each other (26).

It is worth noting that PDiv is not a risk factor for pancreatic adenocarcinoma or TIPMP. Similarly, PDiv has not been identified as a risk factor for neuroendocrine tumor or biliary malignancy (27, 28).

4. Pathogeny of Acute Pancreatitis due to PDiv:

The majority of patients with PDiv remain asymptomatic. As a result, there are still many controversies concerning the imputability of PDiv in the inflammatory pathology of the pancreas.

One of the theories reported in the literature is that of the "dominant duct syndrome" (29, 30) described as follows: the fact that a longer and wider dorsal duct opens through a relatively stenosed and small minor papilla may lead to a drainage mismatch between pancreatic secretion debit and outflow obstruction. The result is increased intraductal pressures and distension of the dorsal canal, leading possibly to abdominal pain and even acute pancreatitis.

Manometric studies on PDiv have shown increased pressures in the dorsal canal and minor papilla compared to those in the ventral canal and major papilla (31). However, the majority of patients with a PDiv and a dilated dorsal duct are asymptomatic. This suggests a low correlation between obstruction and symptoms (32, 33).

The occurrence of these clinical manifestations in adulthood suggests an association of this pancreatic malformation (PDiv) with a newly acquired pathological event. This is usually an organic stenosis of the minor papilla, probably related to the phenomena of ageing (30, 34). Indeed, in the series of Warshaw et al. (30), concerning 88 patients with symptomatic PDiv (without chronic pancreatitis lesions), intraoperative exploration had noted in 75% of cases an exclusively mucosal stenosis of the accessory papilla.

Furthermore, Bertin et al. (35) found that the frequency of pancreas divisum is the same in patients with idiopathic pancreatitis as in control subjects. This means that pancreas divisum (on its own) is probably not a cause of pancreatitis. So, the authors hypothesized that the PDiv may act as a co-factor in patients with genetic pancreatitis, particularly those with CFTR (cystic fibrosis transmembrane conductance regulator gene) mutations.

Other observational studies of patients with idiopathic recurrent acute pancreatitis and chronic pancreatitis (CP) showed that the rates of acute pancreatitis relapses in patients with PDiv and in the normal population were similar (36-38).

Furthermore, in contrast to the study by Bertin et al. other studies have shown a high prevalence of complete or incomplete PDiv in adults (39-41) and children (42) with idiopathic recurrent acute pancreatitis and chronic pancreatitis (CP). This argues for the pathogenicity of PDiv.

The finding of limited morphological changes in the dorsal pancreas during pancreatitis outbreaks in patients with PDiv is also an argument used by some authors to consider PDiv as a potentially pathological entity (41, 43). Similarly, the results of specific treatments targeting the accessory papilla and dorsal duct were also considered as an argument in favor of the pathogenicity of PDiv (44-51). However, these results were variable and irrational in the studies including patients with PDiv and chronic abdominal pain. This heterogeneity suggests that PDiv does not act as a primary actor in pancreatic disease, but rather as a cofactor that, in association with others, causes pancreatic disease (52). This concept is also based on studies showing that the prevalence of idiopathic recurrent acute pancreatitis and chronic pancreatitis (CP) is up to 50% in children and adults with PDiv when it is associated with certain genetic mutations such as the mutation of the serine protease inhibitor Kazal type 1 (SPINK1) gene, the cystic fibrosis transmembrane conductance regulator (CFTR) gene, or the chymotrypsin C gene (CTRC) (35, 53-58).

On the other hand, a recent international multicentric study (59) of a large, globally phenotyped pediatric population (INSPPIRE cohort) showed that children with PDiv:

- did not have a higher incidence of SPINK1, CFTR, CTRC mutations than those without PDiv
- had a lower risk of PRSS1 (serine protease 1 gene) mutations or family history of pancreatitis.
- Had a greater risk of hypertriglyceridemia.

So, the study concluded that PDiv is probably a risk factor for idiopathic recurrent acute pancreatitis and chronic pancreatitis regardless of genetic factors. This study showed also that PDiv reduces the trigger threshold of acute pancreatitis caused by alcohol, drugs, and trauma as suggested by the study of Adike et al. (60).

In short, the imputability of the pancreas divisum in the genesis of (pancreatic) clinical manifestations remains a controversial issue to date.

5. Symptomatology

A minor part (only 5%) of patients with PDiv are symptomatic. Three clinical presentations are then possible:

- Pancreatic-like chronic abdominal pain: This concerns 51% of patients with PDiv. In this case, there is no serum elevation of pancreatic enzymes or morphological changes of the pancreas (30).
- Authentic acute pancreatitis: Complications such as ductal lesions, pancreatic necrosis and pseudocysts are possible. This concerns 25% to 50% of patients with PDiv (61-63). It is worth noting that there is no relationship between either the severity or the incidence of acute pancreatitis and the complete or incomplete nature of the PDiv (64).
- Chronic pancreatitis of the dorsal pancreas depending on the dorsal duct: Associated comorbidities such as exocrine and endocrine pancreatic insufficiency, metabolic disorder and chronic abdominal

pain are relatively common. This concerns 25% of patients with PDiv. It may be chronic obstructive or calcifying pancreatitis with however the same prevalence and the same clinical presentation as for the general population (65).

Some very rare complications of the pancreas divisum have also been reported: these are pancreatic pseudocysts (66), pancreatic abscesses (67), and pancreatic hemorrhage from the dorsal duct (68).

6. Imaging and Diagnostic Modalities

6.1. Abdominal CT Scan

Abdominal CT scanning with medium contrast injection can identify the anatomical variants of the pancreatic duct but with a low sensitivity of 50-60% (69). This is all the more difficult as the ductal system is concealed by pancreatic disease such as acute or chronic pancreatitis and their complications.

In the other hand, when the ducts are visible, the sensitivity of this imaging modality rises approximatively to 83%. The CT-scan would then show the dorsal duct passing forward and upward of the bile duct at the head of the pancreas and ends separately at the minor papilla. The ventral duct, which is small and distinct, ends into the major papilla with the choledocus (70).

The dynamic Ct-scan with Secretin provocation may increase the visibility of the pancreatic ducts with a sensitivity of around 83%, apart from situations with pancreatic complications (71).

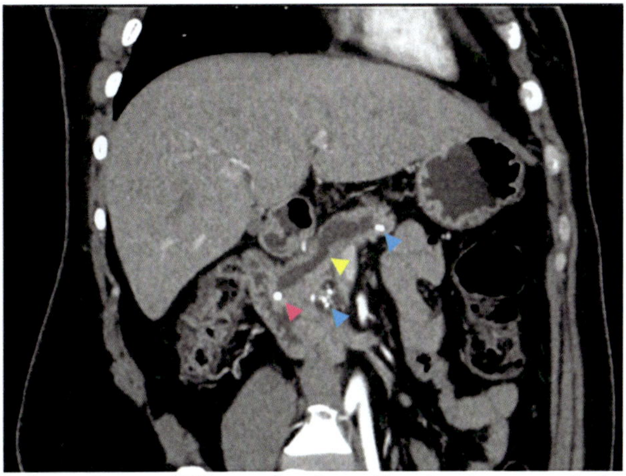

Figure 2-3: Coronal view of CT-scan showing a dilated main pancreatic duct (yellow arrow head). This is the dorsal pancreatic duct draining alone (not in conjunction with common bile duct) into the minor papilla (pink arrow head) where a pancreatic stone is blocked. There is also some pancreatic calcification (blue arrow heads). All these findings are highly suggestive of pancreas divisum with chronic pancreatitis.

6.2. Magnetic Resonance Cholangiopancreatography (MRCP)

The MRCP is the best (non-invasive) imaging for the positive diagnosis of PDiv. It provides a fine map of the pancreatic and bile ducts. Acquisitions are made by magnetic resonance in axial sections with sagittal and frontal reconstructions, with T2-weighted images and according to two types of sequences (34):

- HASTE sequence (Half-Fourier acquisition with single-shot turbo spin echo): axial section allowing excellent visualization of fluid structures.
- RARE sequence (Half-Fourier rapid acquisition with relaxation enhancement) allowing to visualize the common bile duct and the pancreatic ducts in a single image.

On the axial, coronal or 3D sections, this examination shows "the crossing sign": this means that the dorsal (main) pancreatic duct ends in the accessory papilla, pre-crossing the choledocus which ends into the duodenum at the level of the major papilla (Figure 2-4). The ventral pancreatic duct ends also at the level of the major papilla. The description of the ducts' anatomy is then similar to that of the CT-scan.

According to recent meta-analyses and systematic reviews (72-74), MRCP has a sensitivity of 50-70% and of 83-86% after Secretin intravenous injection. It has a specificity of 97-99% (with Secretin injection). Indeed, although the positive predictive value of Secretin is lower in patients suffering from chronic pancreatitis and exocrine pancreatic insufficiency, the contribution of MRCP images with Secretin injection is higher than those without Secretin stimulation.

The cystic dilatation of the terminal portion of the dorsal pancreatic duct next to its junction with the minor papilla is called "Santorinicele". It may also be shown by MRCP with Secretin injection (S-CPRM) (75, 76).

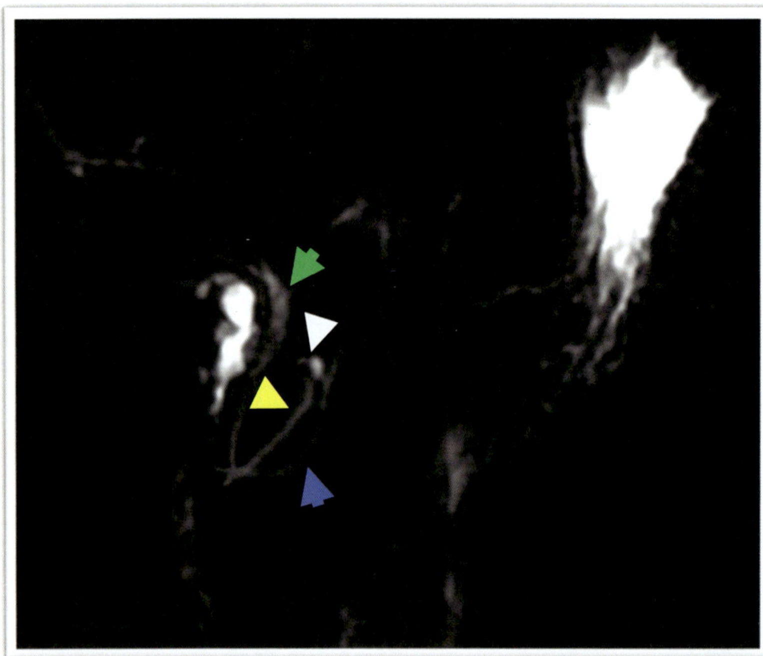

Figure 2-4: MRCP showing an incomplete pancreas divisum. The main pancreatic duct (blue arrow) drains into the minor papilla, the ventral duct (arrow in yellow) drains with the common bile duct (arrow in green) into the major papilla. There is also a very fine ductal rudimentary communication between the ventral and dorsal pancreatic ducts (white arrow).

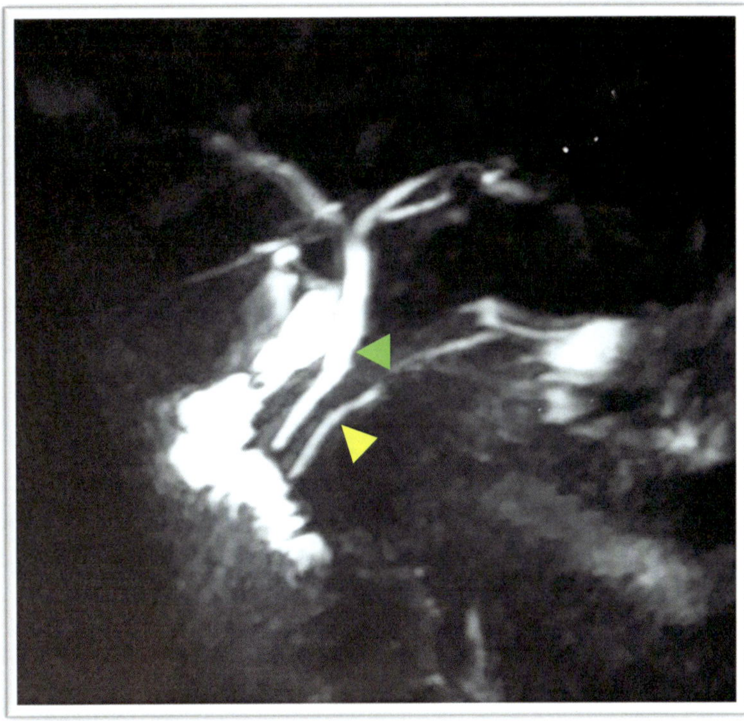

Figure 2-5: MRCP showing an inverted pancreas divisum with a main pancreatic dorsal duct (yellow arrow head) ending into the minor papilla below the major papilla in which ends the common bile duct (green arrow head).

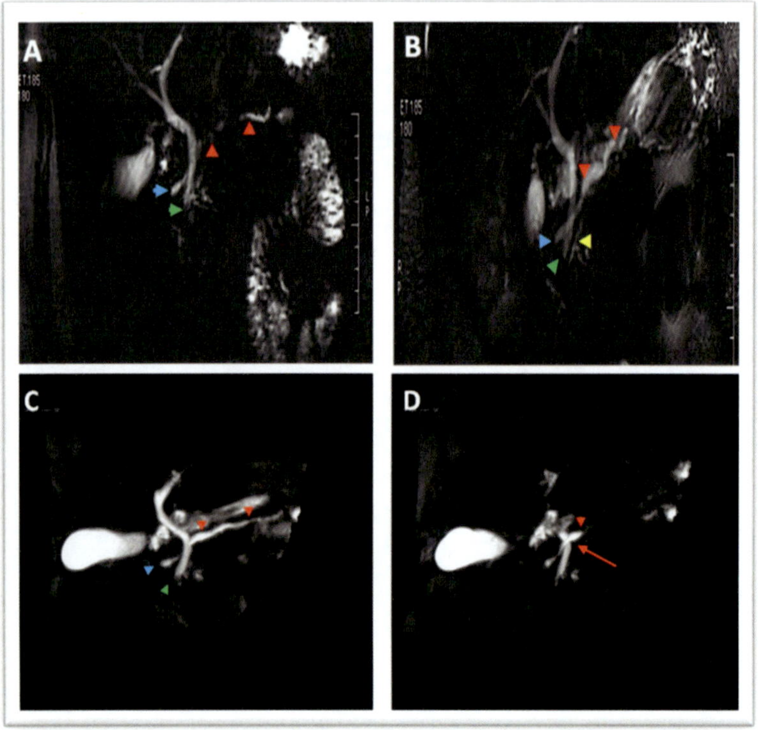

Figure 2-6: Two (A and B) and 3 (C and D) dimensions images of MRCP showing a junction of the main pancreatic duct (heads of red arrows) with the duodenum (blue arrow heads) different from that of the bile duct (green arrow heads). The image D shows a precrossing (red arrow) of the main pancreatic duct with the common bile duct. This is a complete pancreas divisum with an accessory pancreatic duct (yellow arrow head) opening into the major papilla with the common bile duct. Note the irregularities of the main pancreatic duct with images of multiple signal voids related to intra-ductal calcifications (intra ductal stones).

6.3. Endoscopic Ultrasound (EUS)

EUS is a non-invasive imaging that can be useful for the diagnosis of PDiv, but this needs a lot of expertise. Unfortunately, this kind of exploration still not widely available in developing countries.

When the EUS confirms the absence of communication between the ventral and dorsal ducts of the pancreas, it suggests the diagnosis of PDiv

(34). Moreover, the identification of the ventral duct in the corporal-caudal portion of the pancreas rules out PDiv (34, 77).

The EUS Coupled with secretin injection (S-EUS), has shown good diagnostic accuracy in terms of PDiv (70, 78, 79) with a sensitivity of 87-95% (80).

In case of a normal pancreas, the linear sections of EUS would logically show that the ventral duct, the common bile duct and the portal vein are in parallel positions (on a parallel axis). This is called the “stack sign” (77-79).

The absence of the “stack sign” and the ascertainment of the “crossed duct sign” (dorsal duct pre-crosses the common bile duct) is suggestive of pancreas divisum (81).

EUS may also show other signs that allow to rule out a PDiv such as:

- the main pancreatic duct is visualized without interruption: it sinks into the pancreatic parenchyma from the body towards the isthmus and the head of pancreas to end in the major papilla.
- the main pancreatic duct can be traced backwards ("tracing back") from the major papilla towards the body of the pancreas passing through the head and the isthmus of the pancreas. It follows an uninterrupted path from the hypoechoic area (which corresponds to the less fatty ventral pancreas) to the hyperechoic area (which corresponds to the fattier dorsal pancreas) (79, 81).

The tracing may also be done for the dorsal duct which is wider (and the major pancreatic duct) and therefore easily identified nearby the minor papilla in case of PDiv. In this case, it usually follows a straight path, parallel to the splenic vein towards the body and tail of the pancreas (79).

Recent systematic reviews and meta-analyses suggest that S-CPRM is superior to EUS in terms of diagnosing PDiv (73, 74). Factors such as the interposition of gastrointestinal gases and body morphology influenced the sensitivity of EUS and limited its accuracy.

6.4. Does ERCP Contribute to the Diagnosis of PDiv?

The ERCP is considered the gold standard for the diagnosis of PDiv (82, 83) but it is usually performed only if a therapeutic is planned.

ERCP is an invasive examination that requires general anesthesia, exposes the patient to radiation and has its own complications, namely acute pancreatitis, duodenal perforation, acute cholangitis and bleeding.

Given all these ERCP drawbacks on the one hand and the performances of the MRCP or S-MRCP (which is a non-invasive imaging) on the other hand, the latter became the reference investigation for the diagnosis of PDiv.

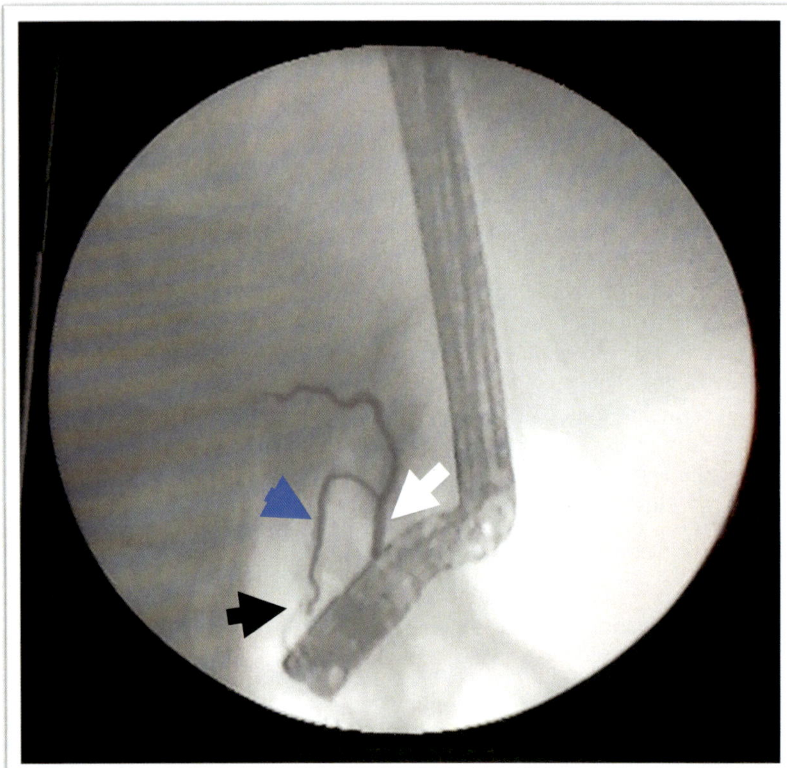

Figure 2-7: ERCP with opacification through the major papilla (arrow in black) showing a communication between the ventral (blue arrow) and the dorsal ducts. The latter is the main pancreatic duct (arrow in white) that drains into the minor papilla. This an incomplete pancreas divisum.

7. Treatment

7.1. Aims and Principles

Treatment of PDiv is restricted to symptomatic patients only. Asymptomatic patients with incidental diagnosis of PDiv do not require further diagnostic investigation or any therapeutic management.

For symptomatic patients with PDiv, the choice of the treatment modality depends on the frequency, the duration, and the intensity of the related symptoms or complications.

For patients with acute pancreatitis (and its possible complications) or with chronic pancreatitis (and its possible comorbidities), a thorough investigation of the underlying etiologies of pancreatic disease should be conducted. This investigation may comprehensively include questioning about family and personal history, lifestyle habits and history of any medication, radiological and biological examinations, genetic testing, and metabolic causes.

Therapeutic management should be considered for patients with recurrent flare-ups of acute pancreatitis regardless of its severity or for those with a single acute pancreatitis severe flare-up without any other obvious cause than PDiv.

Therapeutic management should also be considered in patients with chronic pancreatitis if an obvious manageable target has been identified, i.e., pancreatic stone, dorsal duct stenosis or dilation.

The main principle of symptomatic PDiv treatment is to remove the obstruction particularly at the level of the minor papilla so as to facilitate the pancreatic juice flow along the dorsal duct. This would lower the intraductal pressure and then prevents increased pain and possible flare-ups of acute pancreatitis. This can be done either endoscopically or surgically depending on the patient's profile and the medical team expertise.

7.2. Non Interventional Treatment

This therapeutic option can be considered for patients with moderate symptoms of pancreatic-like abdominal pain without radiological features of chronic pancreatitis.

In this situation, the management is rather conservative, oriented towards symptom management based on non-narcotic analgesics, anti-spasmodics, anti-cholinergics, a low-fat diet and even pancreatic enzyme supplementation therapy.

7.3. Endoscopic Treatment

Endoscopic treatment includes endoscopic sphincterotomy of the minor papilla (ESm), balloon dilation of the minor papilla, and stenting of the dorsal duct through the minor papilla. It is worth noting that the cannulation techniques of the minor papilla are well described in the literature but need a lot of expertise (84, 85).

Compared to the major papilla, the minor papilla is almost always located in the upper right quadrant of the endoscopist's field of vision with a variable distance between the two orifices (10 to 30 millimeters anteriorly) (Figure 2-8).

The success rate of this endoscopic procedure (ESm) is variable, ranging from 73-83% in some studies (86, 87) to 90-95% for experienced interventionist (36, 43).

The failure of the procedure is usually related to one of the following causes:

- an imperceptible minor papilla.
- a twisted minor papilla due to local inflammation (acute pancreatitis or duodenal peptic ulcer).
- a duodenal diverticulum.
- a malignant cause.
- the endoscopist is unable to approach the minor papilla from an adequate angle.

However, there are some technical tricks that would help the endoscopist to identify the minor papilla when it is not clearly visualized. For example:

- Intravenous injection of secretin may stimulate pancreatic exocrine function and pancreatic secretion through the minor papilla. The latter would then become prominent and easily spotted (88).
- Chromoendoscopy or spraying the duodenal mucosa with dilute Methylene Blue, can help identify the minor papilla. this will draw a clearing of pancreatic secretions marking this papilla. These techniques would be more effective if coupled with secretin injection.
- Injection of Methylene blue into the ventral duct into the major papilla would help identify the minor papilla which should ooze a blue liquid in case of incomplete pancreas divisum because there is a communication between the ventral and dorsal pancreatic ducts (89).

The ESm is a procedure that has been shown to be effective in patients with symptomatic PDiv (47, 49, 50, 90). However, the risk of complications is similar to that of endoscopic sphincterotomy of the major papilla (ESM) with the same risk factors for post-ERCP acute pancreatitis, namely young age, female gender, previous attack(s) of post-ERCP acute pancreatitis and absence of chronic pancreatitis (91, 92).

In the same vein, the secretin provocation would make it easier to locate the minor papilla and therefore minimize the risk of post-ERCP acute pancreatitis.

Temporary, prophylactic pancreatic stenting after ESm has been advocated to reduce the risk of post-ERCP acute pancreatitis (93-95). These temporary stents usually migrate spontaneously from the pancreatic duct into the duodenum after 2 weeks (96). It may also be removed endoscopically if it does not migrate (97, 98).

Intra rectal administration of 100 milligrams of indomethacin before and after the procedure as well as infusion of a Ringer-Lactate solution has also been shown to decrease the risk of post-PRCP acute pancreatitis (99-103).

Balloon dilatation of the minor papillary orifice is also an effective therapeutic endoscopic option (104, 105). It usually needs a pancreatic stent placement after the procedure given the high risk of post-ERCP acute pancreatitis. Nevertheless, balloon papillary dilatation is currently being abandoned by some endoscopic teams due to a high rate of pancreatic trauma (106).

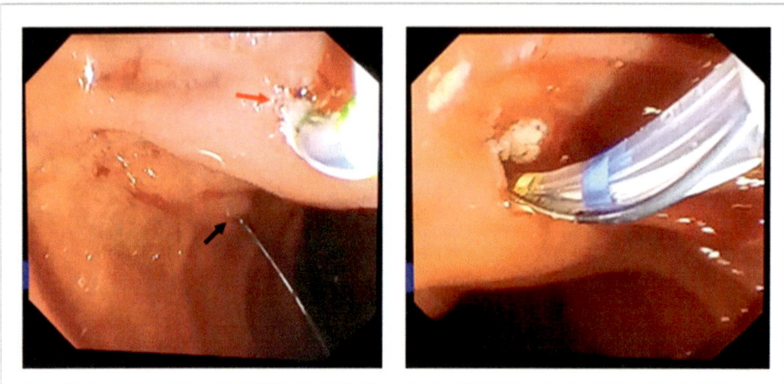

Figure 2-8: Image to the left: Endoscopic view showing the guide wire exiting by the major papilla (arrow in black). It was introduced by the minor papilla (arrow in red). This confirms that there is a communication between the ventral and the dorsal pancreatic ducts. The minor papilla is almost always located in the upper right quadrant of the endoscopist's field of vision anteriorly to the major papilla with a variable distance between the two orifices (10 to 30 millimeters). Image to the right: endoscopic view of an endoscopic sphincterotomy of the minor papilla.

Dorsal pancreatic duct stenting with or without ESm or balloon dilatation can go a long way in getting rid of the PDiv symptoms (45, 46, 48, 51, 86). However, it has its specific complications, namely: prosthesis migration (107), prosthesis occlusion (108), ductal perforation, hemorrhage, acute pancreatitis with possible pseudocyst formation (109), and the development of ductal and/or parenchymal lesions of chronic pancreatitis (110, 111).

The overall incidence of post-ERCP pancreatitis is 10-15% (112, 113).

The effectiveness of the endoscopic treatment is variable and depends mainly on the clinical presentation. This has been proven in multiple studies over the years:

- The results of 4 recent systematic reviews and meta-analyses (6, 114-116) are as following:
  - An average success rate of 62-70%.
  - The optimal response to endoscopic treatment was noted in patients with recurrent acute pancreatitis (76-80%).
  - A lower success rate was observed in patients with chronic pancreatitis (42-69%).

    - The lowest success rate was found in patient with chronic pancreatic-like abdominal pain (33-54%).
- Tierney et al. (117) published a retrospective comparative study in 2020 and found that the group of patients who had 3 or more ERCPs were significantly more likely to require surgery. This study also found that chronic pancreatitis, biliary dilatation and back pain were predictive of poor response to endoscopic treatment should be the indication for surgery after at least one ERCP.
- Boerma et al. (118) consider that only one third of patients with PDiv and chronic pancreatitis improve after pancreatic stenting, one third remain unchanged, and one third will require surgery.

In short, assessment of the response to endoscopic treatment is oftenly limited by the retrospective and uncontrolled nature of the studies reported in the literature (Tables 2-1, 2-2, 2-3 and 2-4). It is currently proven that there is significant variability in patient responses to endoscopic management of symptomatic PDiv. It is also clear that patient response is not solely dependent on its clinical presentation. Indeed, the level of expertise of the endoscopist in ERCP could explain some of this variability, but this has not been documented yet in most published studies.

In addition, special attention should be paid to two other important key points:

- First, there is no consistency between definitions of response to treatment
- Second, the success criteria for endoscopic treatment must be standardized for each group of patients (for those with recurrent acute pancreatitis, for those with chronic pancreatitis and for those with chronic abdominal pain) in order to better assess the success rate by indication, the duration of follow-up and the incidence of post-ERCP complications.

Table 2-1: Definitions of response to endoscopic treatment of symptomatic PDiv (part 1)

The definition includes an objective detection of at least one episode of acute pancreatitis (After a first ERCP attempt)			
Author	**Country**	**Study**	**Definition of response to endoscopic treatment**
McCarthy et al (84)	USA	Prospective	Reduction in the frequency of flare-ups and emergency room visits.
Lehman et al (47)	USA	Prospective	Decrease in at least two of the following criteria: use of narcotics, number of episodes of pancreatitis, number of emergency room visits and/or hospitalizations for abdominal pain.
Chacko et al (45)	USA	Retrospective	For patients with recurrent acute pancreatitis: Reduction $\geq$50% in the annual number of pancreatitis episodes. For patients with chronic pancreatitis or chronic abdominal pain: Reduction $\geq$50% in pain score, use of narcotics, annual number of emergency room visits and/or hospitalizations for abdominal pain.
Lans et al (46)	USA	Prospective	Reduction $\geq$50% in annual number of emergency room visits and/or hospitalizations for abdominal pain, annual number of pancreatitis episodes, Improvement $\geq$50% in patient perception on a visual analogue scale.

Table 2-2: Definitions of response to endoscopic treatment of symptomatic PDiv (part 2)

The definition includes an objective detection of at least one episode of acute pancreatitis (After a first ERCP attempt)			
Author	**Country**	**Study**	**Definition of response to endoscopic treatment**
Mariani et al (113)	Italy	Retrospective	No recurrence of pancreatitis at follow-up
Kwan et al (50)	Australia	Retrospective	No recurrence of pancreatitis at follow-up.
Ertan et al (86)	USA	Prospective	Disappearance of symptoms with no reports of hospitalizations and/or emergency room visits for abdominal pain or recurrent pancreatitis during follow-up.
Jacob et al (87)	USA	Retrospective	No recurrence of pancreatitis or pancreatic-like pain.

Table 2-3: Definitions of response to endoscopic treatment of symptomatic PDiv (part 3)

The definition depends on the patient's perception of the pain and/or the effectiveness of the treatment			
Author	**Country**	**Study**	**Definition of response to endoscopic treatment**
Borak et al (44)	USA	Retrospective	Clinical improvement without the use of narcotics after initial ERCP.
Gerke et al (90)	USA	Retrospective	Disappearance of symptoms or minimal symptoms (≤ 2 on a visual analogue scale of 0-10) after first ERCP with disappearance of symptoms after second ERCP.
Heyries et al (48)	France	Retrospective	Non recurrence or reduction in the perception of acute pancreatitis and disappearance or fewer episodes of pain requiring analgesics.
Boerma et al (118)	Netherlands	Retrospective	No symptoms during follow-up.
Kozarek et al (110)	USA	Retrospective	Patient reporting of a significant response (overall improvement) after a first ERCP
Siegel et al (51)	USA	Prospective	Improvement of all symptoms associated with pancreatitis.

Table 2-4 : Definitions of response to endoscopic treatment of symptomatic PDiv (part 4)

The definition based on the use of a treatment or a need of intervention			
Author	**Country**	**Study**	**Definition of response to endoscopic treatment**
Benage et al (43)	USA	Retrospective	No need for any treatment or intervention after first ERCP.
The definition of response to endoscopic treatment is not well specified			
Author	**Country**	**Study**	**Definition of response to endoscopic treatment**
Yamamoto et al (104)	Japan	Retrospective	"Improvement of symptoms", no other criteria.

7.4. Surgical treatment

Surgical sphincterotomy of the minor papilla (49), as well as surgical sphincteroplasty (33, 119), are two valid options and well-described techniques, which have shown comparable efficiency in symptoms' relief. The best success rate was noted especially in patients suffering of recurrent acute pancreatitis related to PDiv.

All surgical techniques targeting the minor papilla have variable treatment response depending on the clinical presentation. For example, a systematic review published in 2009 (6) reported the following surgical outcomes that are approximately similar to endoscopic treatment results:

- A mean success rate of 75%.
- The maximum efficacy was observed in patients with recurrent acute pancreatitis (83%).
- Lower efficacy in the chronic pancreatitis group (67%).
- The lowest success rate in patients with chronic pancreatic abdominal pain (52%).
- The patients underwent a 6 to 12 months follow-up and a minimal 50 months follow-up period in the majority of studies.

In addition, the comparison of patients with 3 different subtypes of PDiv (complete PDiv, incomplete PDiv and isolated dorsal duct) didn't show any significative difference in clinical presentations and in response to (endoscopic or surgical) treatment rates (6).

Both surgical and endoscopic treatments have shown the same results on symptom relief, but because of higher surgery complication and mortality rates, endoscopic management is considered as the first line treatment. The surgery is therefore restricted for patients in whom cannulation of the minor papilla has failed, or in those with altered anatomy (as gastric bypass...).

It is worth noting that there are limited treatment options for patients with recurrent acute pancreatitis in whom treatment of the minor papilla has unfortunately failed, or who have progressed to chronic pancreatitis. So, in this case, management should aim to control the chronic pancreatitis related symptoms. These treatment options are jejunal feeding to put the pancreatic gland at rest, blockage of the celiac plexus, Somatostatin analogues and intrathecal analgesia by implantable pump (120). Patients with significant dilatation of the dorsal duct may benefit from a latero-lateral pancreaticojejunal anastomosis (Frey or Puestow procedure) (121, 122).

Surgery should be considered in the following situations:

- Failure of endoscopic treatment with symptomatic patients.
- Chronic pancreatitis with local complications such as stenosis of the main bile duct or pancreatic duct.

The surgical strategy aims to treat local complications and to optimize the drainage of the pancreas.

Ferri et al. (112) described in 2019, after a review of the literature from 1990 to 2018, the different techniques and indications of surgical decompression or resection procedures (Figure 2-9). It should be noted that sphincteroplasty, duodenopancreatectomy and pancreatic head resection preserving the duodenum are the most performed techniques.

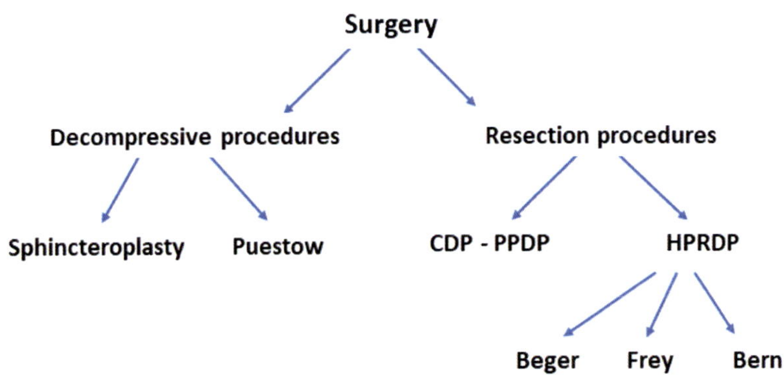

Figure 2-9: Different surgical procedures for the management of the pancreas divisum. CDP-PPDP: Conventional or pylorus preserving duodenopancreatectomy. HPRDP: Head pancreatic resection with duodenal preservation.

7.4.1. Decompressive surgical procedures

7.4.1.1. Trans duodenal sphincteroplasty

Trans duodenal sphincteroplasty of the minor papilla is one of the most used techniques. After duodenotomy (Figure 2-10), the small caruncle is intubated with a lacrimal tube and gradually dilated. This allows to perform a pancreatography so as to eliminate a possible ductal obstruction. Then, the papilla is transected broadly and the edges of the dorsal pancreatic duct are sutured to the duodenal mucosa. Usually, a pancreatic stent is installed for the first 2-3 weeks in order to avoid postoperative stenosis by oedema or early fibrosis (123). As a final step, a cholecystectomy should be performed.

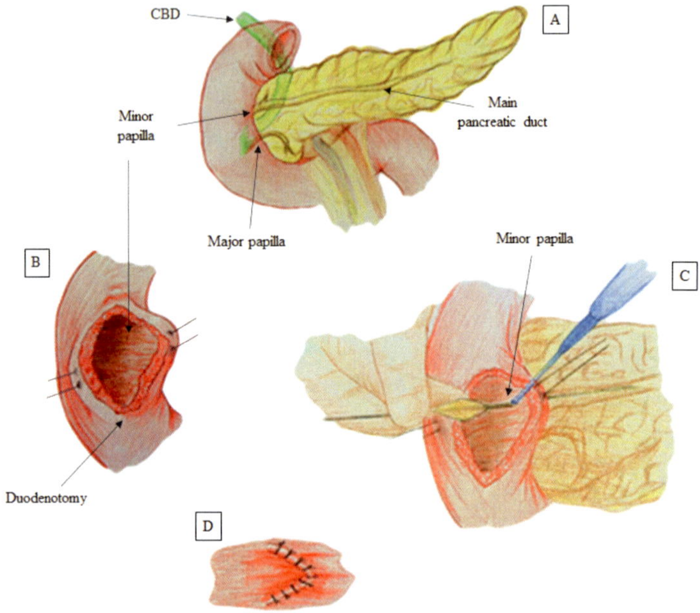

Figure 2-10: Minor papilla trans duodenal sphincteroplasty. A: Anatomical illustration of main pancreatic duct and both major and minor papillas. B: Longitudinal duodenotomy exposing the minor papilla. C: Cannulation of the main pancreatic duct with a lacrymal probe and sphincterotomy of the minor papilla. D: Suture of the main pancreatic duct mucos to the duodenal mucos with separated stitches using a 5/0 absorbable thread.

Sphincteroplasty was the main surgical treatment for pancreas divisum before the era of endoscopic drainage (124) but, its current indications have become limited. It is obviously a very complex technique which, despite its parenchyma-sparing virtue. In addition, it has a low success rate (63%). Thus, and according to Ferri et al., it should not be considered as the first option in the surgical treatment of pancreas divisum (112).

7.4.1.2. Puestow procedure

When the parenchymal and ductal lesions of chronic pancreatitis cause ductal obstruction and dilatation of the main pancreatic duct, a longitudinal lateral pancreaticojejunal anastomosis can be performed (Figure 2-11). Schnelldorfer (125) reports 21 cases of pancreas divisum with chronic pancreatitis that were treated using the Puestow procedure with a 90% success rate.

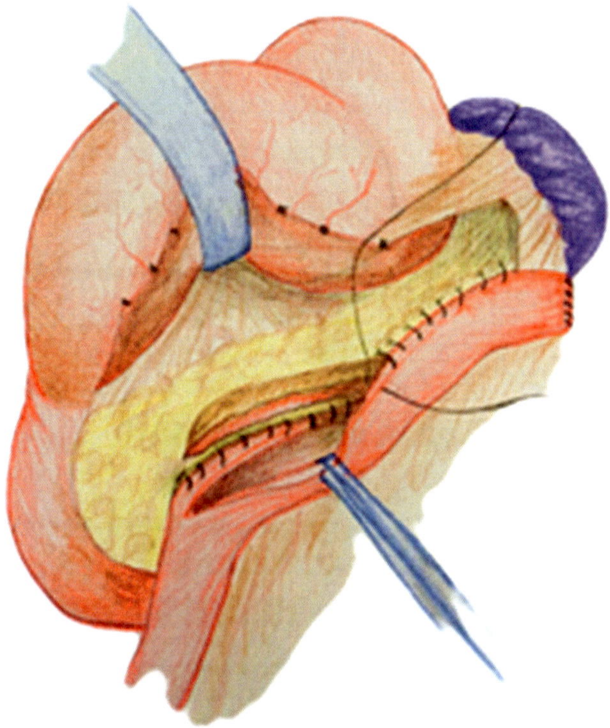

Figure 2-11: Puestow procedure: Latero-lateral pancreatojejunal anastomosis.

7.4.2. Resection procedures

Studies comparing resection procedures for the treatment of pancreas divisum are currently insufficient to identify the best technique. Of all the surgical techniques, duodenopancreatectomy – with or without preservation of the pylorus – and pancreatic head resection preserving the duodenum are the best known and most widely applied. The success rate varies from 80 to 100% with a complication rate of 0 to 33% (126).

7.4.2.1. Conventional or pylorus preserving duodenopancreatectomy (CD-PPDP) (Figure 2-12):

The pylorus preservation technique is less aggressive. When performed in expert pancreatic surgery centers, an operative mortality of 2-5% is reported, with a success rate of 80% in the treatment of PDiv (127).

7.4.2.2. Head pancreatic resection with duodenal preservation (HPRDP) (Figure 2-12):

Since duodenopancreatectomy has a high complication rate and a significant mortality rate in the treatment of benign disease, more cost-effective resection techniques have been proposed, with the aim of minimizing the impact of the surgery and preserving the enteroendocrine axis.

According to Beger et al. (128), the pancreas is transected at the isthmus in front of the portal vein. The pancreatic head is then detached, but not completely removed, thus preserving the duodenum and the deep layer of pancreatic tissue. Reconstruction is then performed with two anastomoses, namely the Wirsungo-jejunal anastomosis and the anastomosis of the pancreatic head with the jejunum in order to drain the remaining parenchyma and to cover the defect of the pancreatic head (Figure 2-12). If necessary, the common bile duct can be drained to avoid an ischemic complication.

Frey et al. (129) described a modified duodenal head resection that represents a hybrid technique between the Beger and Puestow procedures. In Frey's technique, the pancreatic head resection is smaller, and a lateral pancreaticojejunal anastomosis is performed to drain the entire pancreatic duct. This technique is not eligible in the case of a pancreas divisum with chronic pancreatitis and a large inflammatory mass of the head of the pancreas. However, it appears to be advantageous in cases where the inflammatory component is minor and may be suitable for resolving an obstruction in the distal (tail side) pancreatic duct.

In the Bern procedure (130), the excavation of the pancreatic head can be performed in the same way as in the Beger procedure, but the difference is that the pancreas section is not performed in front of the portal vein. The digestive reconstruction can be achieved by a single anastomosis between the excavated pancreatic head and a jejunal loop (Figure 2-12).

This technique is suitable when the inflammatory mass (of the pancreatic head) is not associated with distal pancreatic duct stenosis. In addition, and when necessary, a bilio-enterostomy may be performed.

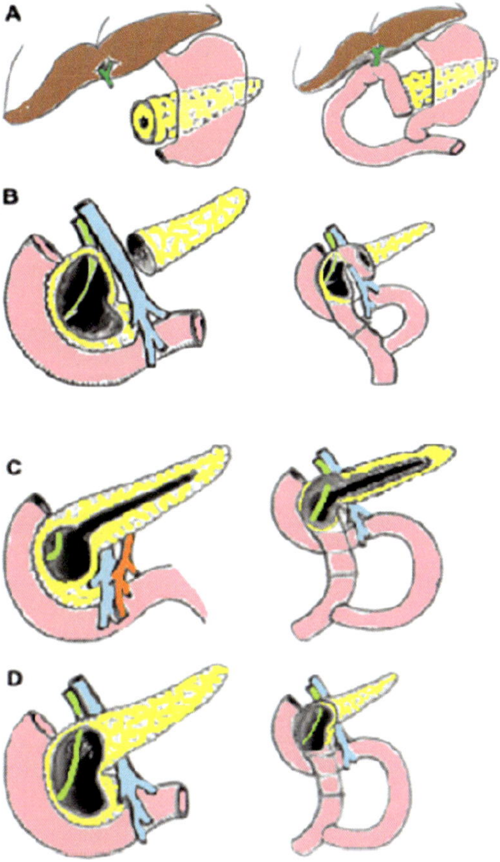

Figure 2-12: Surgical resection procedures.

A: Duodenopancreatectomy. B: Beger technique. C: Frey intervention. D: Bern proceduren. B, C, D: Resection of the head of the pancreas with duodenal preservation.

7.4.2.3. Pancreatic Head Resection with Segmental Duodenal Resection (PHRSD)

Nakao et al. described the Pancreatic Head Resection with Segmental Duodenectomy in 1998 (131). This technique allows a complete resection of the pancreatic head with resection of the second portion of the duodenum (a segmental duodenal resection). This means that minor and major papilla are resection en-bloc with this duodenal segment. The first portion of the duodenum is preserved to maintain the gastroduodenal artery and the anterosuperior pancreaticoduodenal arch. The third and fourth portions of the duodenum are also preserved to maintain the posteroinferior pancreaticoduodenal arch. An end-to-end duodenal anastomosis is then performed in addition to Roux-en-Y hepaticojejunostomy and to a latero-lateral pancreaticojejunostomy (Figure 2-13). Nakao et al. reported 67 cases of head resection with segmental duodenectomy (132) for the treatment of IPMNP (intra papillary mucinous neoplasm of the pancreas). In this study, there was a zero-mortality rate and the fistula rate was 10% and 13% for type A and B fistulas respectively.

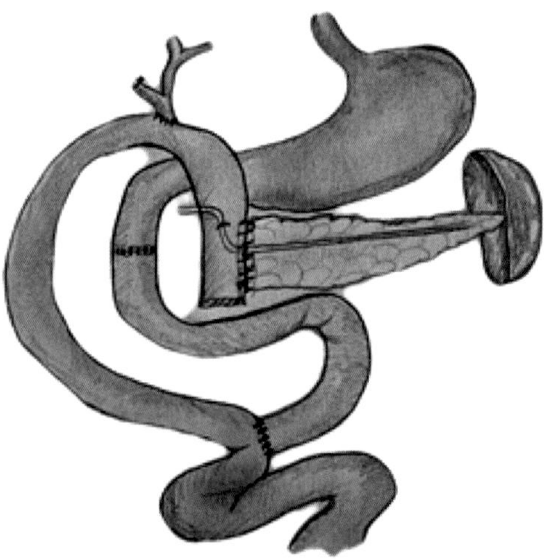

Figure 2-13: Nakao technique.

The Nakao technique should be considered, according to Ferri's team (112), as the first surgical option given its encouraging outcomes on patients with pancreas divisum and chronic pancreatitis.

7.4.2.4. Total dorsal pancreatectomy (TDP)

Total Dorsal Pancreatectomy has been indicated for benign or low-grade dysplastic tumors confined to the dorsal pancreas such as IPMNP or SPPNP (Solid pseudopapillary neoplasm of the pancreas) (133).

In patients with PDiv, the cleavage plane between the dorsal and ventral pancreas may be easily identified at the postero-superior portion of the pancreatic head. Thayer (134) describes this plane as a fibrous septum running anterior to the choledocus and allowing non-bleeding dissection of both segments. The dorsal segment of the pancreas is then removed en-bloc with the minor papilla, the body and the tail of the pancreas. The spleen should be preserved whenever possible.

Table 2-5*:* Outcomes of total dorsal pancreatectomy for pancreas divisum: published case reports.

Auth	Year	Age	Sex	Hist	PF	EI	Di	FU (Ms)
Thayer (134)	2002	71	W	IPMNP	Grade B	-	+	12
Talbot (135)	2005	51	W	IPMNP	-	+	+	76
Scatton (136)	2006	45	M	IPMNP	Grade B	-	+	18
Conci (133)	2018	35	W	SPPNP	-	-	-	120

Auth: Author; **Di:** Diabetes; **EI:** Exocrine insuffisancy; **FU:** Follow-up
Hist: Histology; **PF:** Pancreatic fistula; **Ms:** Months

In short, total dorsal pancreatectomy is a feasible and safe procedure for an isolated lesion of the dorsal pancreas that do not require lymph node resection (Table 2-2).

7.4.2.5. Total pancreatectomy with islet auto-transplantation

Total pancreatectomy with islet auto-transplantation is an emerging and promising option in patients who has not responded to endoscopic treatment, but it is still undergoing validation (137-140).

7.5. Endoscopic Versus Surgical Procedures

The endoscopic and surgical procedures are not easy to perform and still have significant failure rates and require long follow-up.

However, the indication for a therapeutic procedure must be well considered. Indeed, PDiv should only be treated specifically when it is directly responsible for clinical symptoms or complications. Thus, the decision to intervene should only be made after a thorough and repeated clinical, biological, endoscopic and radiological work-up to rule out any other cause of the clinical manifestations (34).

Hafezi et al. (116) published a systematic review of the literature in 2017 that proved surgical treatment of PDiv is superior to the endoscopic approach as follows:

- Symptoms' improvement was significantly greater in patients treated with surgery than in those treated with endoscopy (72% vs. 62.3%).
- The complication rate of endoscopic procedures was significantly higher than that associated with surgery (31.3% vs. 23.8%).
- Finally, the re-intervention rate was significantly higher in patients in the endoscopic treatment group (28.3% vs 14.4%).

However, the appropriate treatment of PDiv depends on many factors and the decision to opt for a surgical or for an endoscopic treatment must be made on a case-by-case basis.

Indications for surgical diversion of the dorsal pancreatic duct or for pancreatic resection are exceptional and should be discussed on a case-by-case basis, mainly in patients with PDiv and chronic pancreatitis and particularly after endoscopic sphincterotomy failure.

In general, endoscopic treatment should be considered as the primary therapeutic approach. Whereas surgery should be an option of a last resort particularly after endo therapy failure (112, 116, 124).

To date, there is no scientific evidence to make clear recommendation for therapeutic management of PDiv. A large-scale randomized trial is then obviously needed to define the best treatment approach for symptomatic PDiv refractory to mini-invasive (endoscopic) management. In addition, the cost-effectiveness of both surgical and endoscopic procedures is of major importance and should also be assessed in a prospective trial.

CHAPTER 3

THE ANNULAR PANCREAS

Annular pancreas is a rare congenital anomaly in which that corresponds to a pancreatic tissue completely or incompletely encircling the second portion of the duodenum.

Annular pancreas results from an abnormal rotation of the ventral pancreatic vestige around the duodenum during embryonic life. This is why the PDiv is more frequently reported in patients with PAn than in the general population, with a concomitance of 29-36% in published literature reviews (16, 17).

The incidence of PAn remains difficult to determine precisely but according to some autopsy series it is about 3 per 20,000 population (16, 19, 141-143).

1. Embryogenesis

The embryogenesis of the annular pancreas remains hypothetical. In 1901, Tieken proposed that the pancreatic ring was the result of the hypertrophy of the pancreatic head tissues (144).

Taking into account the form of the annular duct on pancreatograms, it is currently widely admitted that the annular pancreas derives from the ventral bud of the pancreas during embryogenesis (145, 146). There are then two important theories concerning the development of the annular pancreas (Figure 3-1):

- Lecco et al. (147) suggest that the right bud of the ventral pancreas adheres and anchors in the duodenal wall to form a ring during embryogenic clockwise rotation.
- On the other hand, Baldwin et al. (148) state that the left bud of the ventral pancreas persists and forms a pancreatic ring around the duodenum.

However, several cases reported in the literature cannot be explained by these 2 embryogenic theories (143, 149).

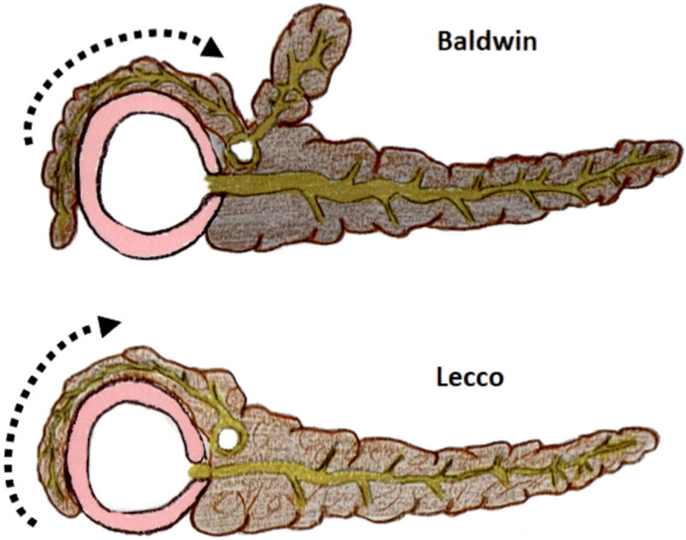

Figure 3-1: Theories of annular pancreas formation.

Annular pancreatic tissue has been shown to be characterized by an abundance of irregularly shaped islets with a very high proportion of PP-positive cells (strongly expressing pancreatic polypeptide), thus proving the ventral origin of the annular pancreas (150, 151).

Yogi et al. established a classification of annular pancreas (152). In this classification, there are 6 types of Annular Pancreas according to the trajectory of the annular duct (Table 3-1):

- The types 1 and 2 are the most common.
- In type 1, the annular duct passes behind the duodenum and opens into the Wirsung.
- In type 2, the annular duct replaces the ventral duct. It emerges from the dorsal duct, then it bypasses the duodenum from front to back and ends into the major papilla.

Table 3-1: Types of annular pancreas according to Yogi classification.

Type	**Schematic illustration**	**Opening site of the annular duct**
I	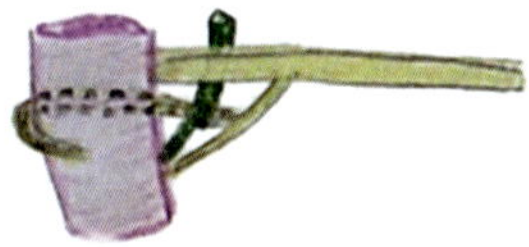	Into the Wirsung from dorsal side
II	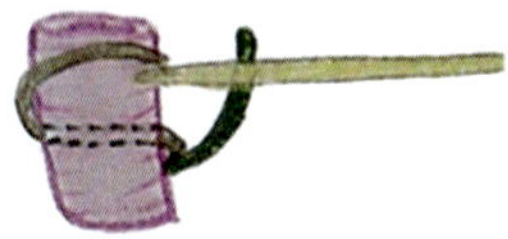	The Wirsung is encircling the duodenum
III	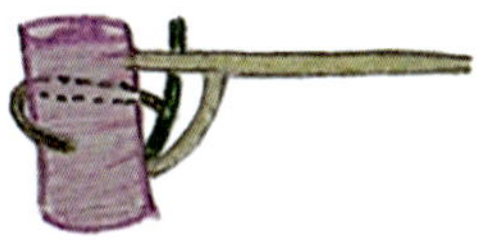	Into the CBD from the dorsal side
IV	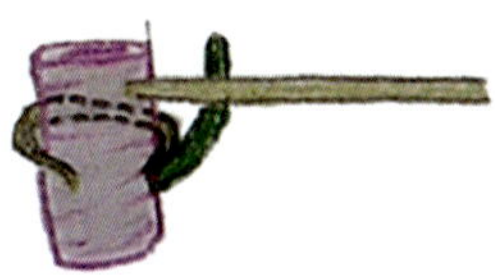	Into the CBD from the dorsal side without the Wirsung
V	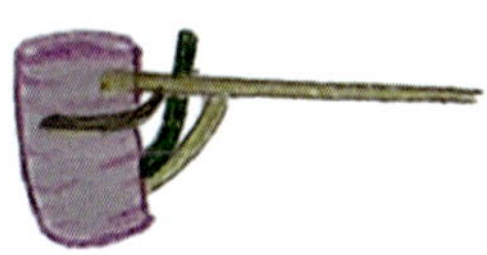	Into the Santorini from the ventral side
VI	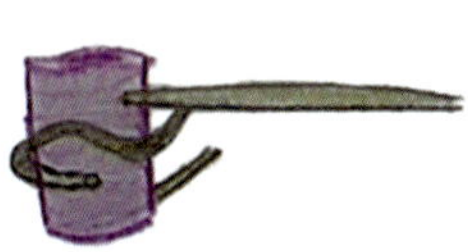	Into the Santorini from the ventral side with a malfusion

Other studies have suggested that more than one mechanism may be involved in the development of the annular pancreas (153). However, over the last three decades, ERCP and MRCP findings suggest that the theories of Lecco and Baldwin are the most plausible (154).

From a molecular standpoint, organogenesis of the pancreas involves the activation/inactivation of components of the Hedgehog signaling pathway. The Hedgehog signaling pathway is a set of genes that code – during embryonic life – for a Hedgehog protein that acts as an intercellular signal controlling cell proliferation and determining cell fate. Dysfunction of the Hedgehog signaling system has been suggested to be a co-factor contributing to the formation of the annular pancreas (155, 156).

From a genetic standpoint, some authors have supported the idea that a dominant (autosomal or X-linked) inheritance may be related to this pancreatic malformation (157-159). Documented family history of annular pancreas cases indicate that genetic inheritance (autosomal dominant or X-linked dominant) is indeed a cause of this pancreatic anomaly. However, obviously many cases of familial annular pancreas go undetected because they remain asymptomatic and may only be discovered at autopsy or incidentally during imaging or surgery done for other purposes. Thus, the genetic basis of a familial form of annular pancreas cannot be ruled out. This will only be duly proven with large studies (particularly autopsy ones) with much more cases of annular pancreas.

Histologically, two forms of annular pancreas can be distinguished: an intramural form in which the pancreatic tissue is interposed between the muscle fibers of the duodenal wall with small pancreatic ducts that drain into the duodenum, and an extramural form, where the annular duct surrounds the duodenum and joins the main pancreatic duct.

2. Clinical Presentation

Annular pancreas is usually, but wrongly, considered a disease of early childhood. In fact, it is diagnosed with almost equal frequency in children and adults. Based on observations at a pediatric center and at an adult pancreaticobiliary center, Zyromski (16) hypothesized not only that annular pancreas encompasses a spectrum of diseases (and of clinical evolution) but also that the pathological processes affecting children are radically different from those in adults. In fact, with a large series of 103 patients with annular pancreas (48 children and 55 adults), Zyromski (16) demonstrated clinical differences between children and adults: all children presented with duodenal obstruction whereas adults had less difficulty with duodenal obstruction, rather they had a much more complex pancreaticobiliary pathology. The study also highlights two other important findings:

- Firstly, the annular pancreas is often associated with other congenital diseases in children, although the pancreas divisum is present in 29% of adults. The most common chromosomal anomaly associated with annular pancreas in children is the trisomy 21.
- Secondly, a significant proportion of adults with annular pancreas (24%) develop neoplasia mainly pancreato-biliary ones (11%). However, some associated congenital anomalies (to annular pancreas) were also reported in adults. The most common are digestive malrotation, duodenal diaphragm and Shatzki's ring were the most common anomalies.

Several publications also reported some other associated cancers with annular pancreas in adults. These are breast cancer, prostate cancer, hematological cancer, colic adenocarcinoma, ovarian cancer, lung cancer and melanoma (160, 161). Thus, close monitoring of patients with annular pancreas is mandatory for early diagnosis of these possible neoplasia (162).

In general, children with annular pancreas present with signs of obstruction of the upper gastro-intestinal tract such as early postprandial vomiting, abdominal distension, and food intolerance. This clinical presentation needs usually imaging as abdominal X-ray, esophageal transit, or abdominal ultrasound for initial diagnostic guidance. Prenatal diagnosis is also possible thanks to prenatal ultrasound that may suggest in 56% of cases the diagnosis of fetal duodenal obstruction related to an annular pancreas. This diagnostic presumption is supported by the presence of a hydramnios (19).

In contrast, the main clinical sign of annular pancreas in adults is abdominal pain (75%) whereas, only 24% would have symptoms related to gastrointestinal obstruction such as postprandial fullness, vomiting, upper gastro intestinal bleeding (secondary to peptic ulceration), and rarely a jaundice related to a biliary obstruction. In addition, 22% of adults with annular pancreas would have an acute or a chronic pancreatitis. This is possibly due to the relatively frequent association with the pancreas divisum (29%). Acute pancreatitis is the second most common clinical presentation of the annular pancreas in adults. Then, duodenal obstruction comes third.

Nagpal et al. (163) found that 60% of adults with annular pancreas are actually asymptomatic with incidental diagnosis of this anomaly.

3. Imaging

The diagnosis of annular pancreas is usually made during radiological investigations of symptomatic patients. But, the diagnosis of this pancreatic anomaly may also incidental. Drey (164) in 1957 suggested a clinical classification of this entity into neonatal, pediatric, asymptomatic adult and symptomatic adult types.

3.1. Annular Pancreas in Neonates and Infants

In symptomatic neonates, ultrasound or plain abdominal radiographs can detect this anomaly by showing the classic double bubble sign indicating some degree of duodenal obstruction.

Patients in this age group who are suspected of having partial or complete duodenal obstruction usually require surgery during which the diagnosis of annular pancreas is confirmed.

Prenatal diagnosis of annular pancreas has also been reported by some authors (165-168) using ultrasound that may show direct signs as hyperechoic pancreatic tissue encircling the duodenum or indirect signs as hydramnios (157).

Yang et al. (169), published in 2019 an ultrasound study of 28 newborns with annular pancreas. They found that an acute angle of 40.7° between the pre-stenotic and post-stenotic duodenal wall, as well as an "S" sign formed by the pylorus, bulb, pre-stenotic and post-stenotic duodenum, allows the diagnosis of annular pancreas with a sensitivity of 100%, specificity of 97.1%, positive predictive value of 96.6%, and negative predictive value of 100%.

3.2. The Upper GI Series

The upper GI series may show indirect signs of D2 (descending duodenum) stricture (or obstruction) by a subtraction image and upstream distension.

3.3. Duodenoscopy and ERCP

Gromski et al. (19) detailed in 2018 the endoscopic and pancreatographic aspects of annular pancreas in 46 patients as follows:

- Fibroscopy can show duodenal stricture or annulus in 87% of patients. But gastric retention is rarely observed. Two phenotypes of annular pancreas seem possible: the first where the ring constricts totally the duodenum causing gastric stasis, the second where the annular ring is relatively loose or incomplete.
- The minor papilla position beside the annular stricture was also specified: it may be proximal (37%) or distal (6%) to the stricture or

located on the stricture itself (31%). The latter position is obviously more difficult to catheterize. Exceptionally, the minor papilla is located at the level of the junction duodenal bulb to the second portion of the duodenum, far from the pancreatic annulus (19).

Despite the technical difficulties (duodenal deformity and position of the minor papilla), ERCP can be easily performed. It may show signs suggestive of chronic pancreatitis in about one third of patients. These signs are mainly focal stenosis or dilatation of the main pancreatic duct and irregular ductal branches. It is worth noting that these signs of chronic pancreatitis are more frequently reported in patients with a coexisting pancreas divisum (38%) compared to those (28%) with normal pancreas (19).

3.4. CT-Scan and CPRM

Abdominal CT-scan and MRCP should show the pancreatic ring surrounding the totally or partially the second portion of the duodenum in all cases:

- The pancreatic tissue or an annular duct completely surrounding the duodenum is visualized in 2/3 of cases (18) (Figure 3-2).
- In 1/3 of cases, the annulus does not completely surround the duodenum. Thus, the diagnosis of an annular pancreas will be confirmed during ERCP or surgery (18). These cases are considered in radiology as an incomplete annular pancreas.

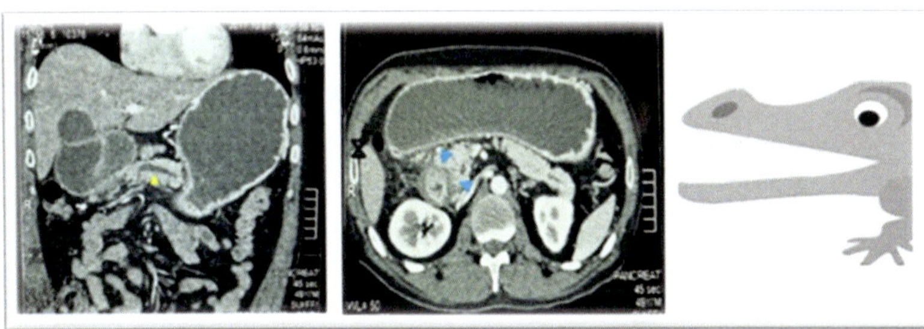

Figure 3-2: Abdominal Ct-scan (with contrast meduim injection) showing a distention of the stomach upstream of a duodenal stenosis (of the second portion of the duodenum), with dilation of the main pancreatic duct (yellow arrow). There is also an antero-lateral and postero-lateral periduodenal extension of the pancreatic parenchyma (blue arrows): this is the "crocodile jaw" sign suggesting the dignosis of an annular pancreas.

The configuration of the pancreatic head surrounding the duodenum may be circular or triangular. The latter corresponds to an incomplete annular pancreas and is recognized in radiology as the "crocodile-jaw sign" (Figure 3-2) (18). The risk of duodenal obstruction due to incomplete annular pancreas (33%) is similar to that of complete one (40%) (18).

Patients who have an incomplete ring of pancreatic tissue around the duodenum on imaging (CT-scan or MRCP) actually have, after ERCP and/or surgical exploration, a thin band of pancreatic tissue that is either peri-duodenal or entirely embedded in the duodenal wall as reported in some publications (18, 170, 171).

The imaging finding of pancreatic tissue extending postero-laterally to the second portion of the duodenum, especially in the setting of upper GI stricture, has a high sensitivity (92%) and 100% specificity for the diagnosis of annular pancreas.

On the other hand, anterolateral extension of the pancreatic tissue is significantly less specific (73%) and slightly more (but not significatively) sensitive (96%) for the diagnosis of annular pancreas (18).

A crocodile jaw configuration of the pancreatic head is highly suggestive of an incomplete annular pancreas.

The best non-invasive investigation to determine the pancreatic ductal configuration and to detect any lesion within the annular duct is the S-MRCP. In fact, Sandrasegaran et al. (18) compared S-CPRM images before and after intravenous injection of secretin in 13 patients and found that the secretin injection significantly increased the sensitivity of the CPRM and showed additional findings such as the presence of an annular pancreas in 2 patients and chronic reshuffle of the annular duct in 3 others.

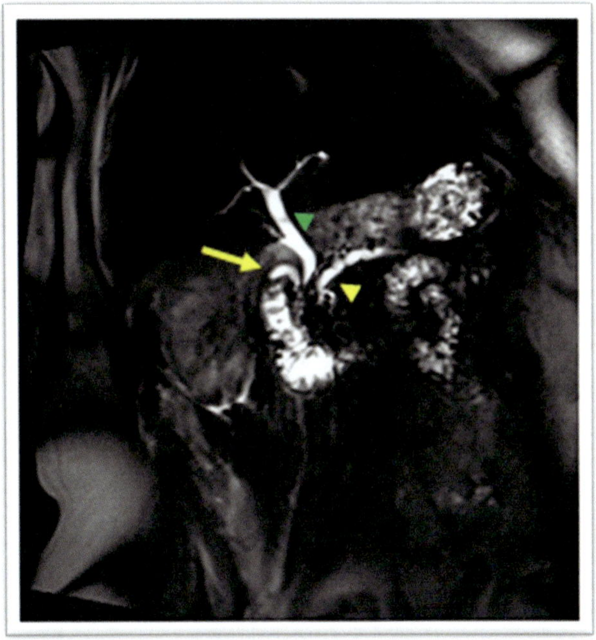

Figure 3-3: Coronal view of MRCP showing a common bile duct (green arrow head) opening separately from the main pancreatic duct (yellow head arrow). There is also a pancreatic duct (yellow arrow) cleaving the second portion of the duodenum: this suggests clearly an annular pancreas.

3.5. Imaging of the Peri-Portal Annular Pancreas

Endoscopic ultrasound (EUS) is the key examination for the diagnosis of periportal annular pancreas. In fact, EUS not only shows the presence of tissue infiltrating the muscle layer of the first portion of the duodenum, but also may allow a biopsy for histological evidence of annular pancreas (161).

The periportal annular pancreas is a congenital variant of the pancreas in which the uncinate process frames the portal vein. Three types of periportal annular have been described:

- Type I in which the main pancreatic duct is located behind the portal vein.
- Type II in which type I is associated with a pancreas divisum.
- Type III in which the main pancreatic duct is located upstream of the portal vein (172, 173).

Although periportal annular pancreas is not associated with an increased risk of pancreaticobiliary disease, it may be misdiagnosed as a mass or tumor enveloping the portal vein.

The prevalence of periportal annular pancreas is estimated at 2.4% (174), but its diagnosis is usually incidental during pancreatic surgery in half of the reported cases (175). Patients with an unrecognized periportal annular pancreas have a 46.7% risk of pancreatic fistula after pancreatic surgery for other cause (175).

4. Treatment

Congenital obstruction of the duodenum in the neonatal period is a relatively common anomaly. It may be a complete or a partial obstruction of an intrinsic or an extrinsic cause. Extrinsic obstruction may be due to several etiologies such as annular pancreas, malrotation and anterior portal vein, all of which are frequently associated with duodenal atresia (176).

Annular pancreas is a congenital anomaly that is usually asymptomatic in adults. However, for symptomatic patients, symptoms are most often present in infancy or the neonatal period (177). More than 40% of cases of annular pancreas are associated with short-term life-threatening duodenal obstruction (178-180). Thus, if diagnosed prenatally, annular pancreas is an important predictor of neonatal gastrointestinal emergencies.

4.1. Treatment of Duodenal Obstruction

For duodenal obstruction associated with an annular pancreas, the best treatment is surgical bypass. This may be done with a gastro-jejunostomy, a duodeno-duodenostomy or a duodenojejunostomy. As the duodeno-duodenal anastomosis is the closest to the anatomy, it is the most recommended for neonates and infants. In addition, a diamond-shaped suture would be the best alternative (176, 181).

The most reported surgical approach is the traditional transverse supra umbilical incision or laparotomy (176). However, laparoscopy is now a mini-invasive surgery that avoids large abdominal incision and associated increased blood loss in addition to an easier and earlier digestive transit recovery (177, 178).

A diamond-shaped duodeno-duodenal anastomosis may also be performed with this minimally invasive approach. This needs a proximal transverse duodenal incision and a distal longitudinal duodenotomy with an incision length of approximately 1 to 1.5 centimeters. The tightness of the anastomosis can be checked by a Methylene Blue test.

Laparoscopy may also reveal other associated gastrointestinal congenital anomalies (even misdiagnosed preoperatively) such as intestinal malrotation, Meckel's diverticulum, duodenal diaphragm or duodenal diverticulum. These anomalies can possibly be treated at the same operative time (181). Thus, and given the high incidence of these associated congenital anomalies (with the annular pancreas), it is imperative that the surgeon carefully explore the rest of the gastrointestinal tract during either open or laparoscopic surgery.

Duodenal obstruction means that the entire jejunum and ileum are decompressed. The absence of air in the bowel downstream of the pancreas is of great benefit when using a laparoscopic approach, as the relatively narrow intra-abdominal space in neonates makes the procedure more difficult and slower than in older children and adults (181).

4.2. Treatment of Acute Pancreatitis

The treatment of acute pancreatitis due to annular pancreas in adults who do not have a duodenal obstruction is still controversial to date.

Most patients with acute pancreatitis are managed conservatively. In general, they do not require surgery solely on the basis of the presence of annular pancreas. However, although the conservative approach provides temporary relief, it does not annihilate the risk of subsequent acute pancreatitis recurrence, chronic pancreatitis or pancreatic malignancy (176).

Surgical resection of the pancreatic ring was initially supported by early studies, but has been abandoned as it has been shown to be associated with an increased risk of complications such as pancreatic fistulas and postoperative acute pancreatitis (146, 163, 164, 182, 183).

Nagpal et al. (163) suggest that the Whipple procedure with pyloric preservation may be considered exceptionally in case of recurrent and crippling acute pancreatitis. It should be decided on a case-by-case basis.

CHAPTER 4

AGENESIS OF THE DORSAL PANCREAS

The ADP is an extremely rare congenital anomaly, which results from the embryological failure of the dorsal pancreatic bud to form the body and the tail segments of the pancreas. It may be asymptomatic and it can be detected incidentally on imaging (184, 185).

1. Embryogenesis

ADP is caused embryologically by either the absence or the involution of the dorsal bud. There are actually 2 types of ADP: the partial and the complete ones.

In complete ADP, the minor papilla, the Santorini duct, and the 3 distal potions of the pancreas (the isthmus, the body and the tail) are absent.

In contrast, the minor papilla, the Santorini duct and a variable portion of the body of the pancreas are present in partial agenesis (185, 186).

2. Epidemiology

In the literature, the study of ADP has been limited to case reports. This is due to the extreme rarity of this condition. Therefore, the incidence of ADP is still unknown. Since its first description by Heiberg in 1911 (187) and until 2008, Schnedl (186) reported 53 cases, but between 2008 and 2015, Cienfuegos J.A (188) reported 53 other patients including 7 children and 46 adults. The increasing number of cases reported in recent years is certainly due to the advent of new imaging techniques.

The ADP has been reported in both children and adults. It may be associated with an autosomal dominant mutation in the hepatocyte nuclear factor 1B (HNF1B) gene, although it seems to be sporadic in the majority of reported cases (189-191).

3. Clinical Presentation

The clinical presentation of the ADP is highly variable: it may be asymptomatic and incidentally discovered on imaging, surgery or autopsy. It may also be diagnosed during assessment of a pancreatic adenocarcinoma (186, 192).

The diagnosis of the ADP requires confirmation of the absence of the isthmus, body, tail and dorsal pancreatic duct by either ERCP or MRCP (188).

As most Langerhans islets are located in the tail of the pancreas, abdominal pain and type II diabetes are the most common clinical manifestations of endocrine insufficiency (186, 193-195). Weight loss has also been reported in patients with ADP and it is thought to be due to steatorrhea (exocrine insufficiency) as well as insulinopenia.

The association of the ADP with cystic neoplasms of the pancreas, chronic non-alcoholic pancreatitis and possibly pancreatic ductal adenocarcinoma has also been reported (192). Other authors have reported an association of ADP with ampullary adenocarcinoma and IPMNP (196, 197).

The enlargement of the residual pancreas and acute recurrent pancreatitis have also been reported as clinical presentation of the ADP (198). From a physio pathological standpoint, 2 factors lead to recurrent acute pancreatitis: the first is the dysfunction of the sphincter of Oddi, and the second is the intraductal hyper pressure that is related to the hypertrophy of the ventral bud of the pancreas and to the compensatory pancreatic enzymes' hypersecretion (186).

Some malformative anomalies (199) have been reported to be associated with the ADP such as visceral heterotaxy syndrome (intestinal malrotation, polysplenia and congenital heart disease as tetralogy of Fallot, aorta coarctation).

4. Imagery

Cystic lesions in the residual pancreas may be misdiagnosed as SPPNP, especially if there are calcifications within the cyst (200).

The pseudocyst is thought to be the result of recurrent acute pancreatitis (even with subclinical episodes). The calcifications within the pseudocyst most likely to be indicate chronic pancreatitis (200).

Both ERCP and MRCP may confirm the diagnosis of the ADP by showing the anatomy of the pancreatic ducts. However, ERCP remains an invasive and operator-dependent procedure. On the other hand, MRCP is a non-invasive examination that doesn't need any pancreatic duct cannulation as in ERCP (185).

Actually, the CT-scan is the first-line imaging for pancreatic abdominal pain, but its findings must be combined to those of the ERCP or the MRCP so as to establish the diagnosis of the ADP (Figures 4-1 and 4-2) (185).

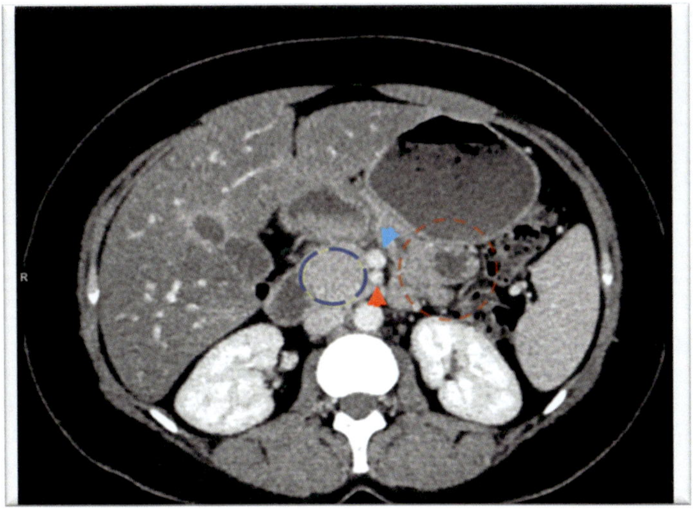

Figure 4-1: Abdominal CT-scan showing corporeo-caudal agenesis of the pancreas (space in red dotted line occupied by small intestine loops). The pancreas is limited to its cephalic portion (blue dotted area). Blue (vein) and red (artery) arrowheads show superior mesenteric vessels.

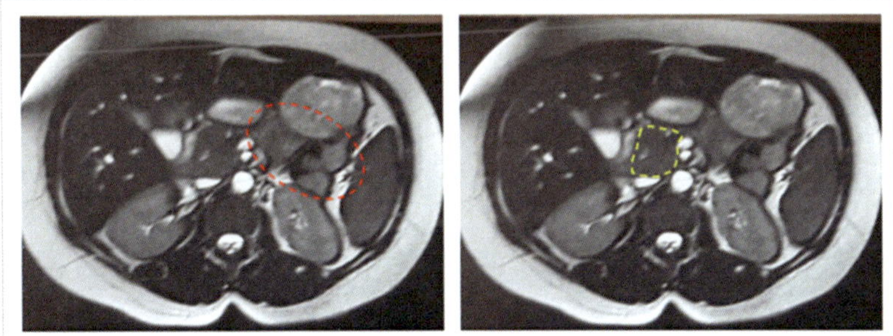

Figure 4-2: MRCP showing corporeal caudal agenesis of the pancreas (red dotted area). The bed of the agennesic pancreas is occupied by small intestine loops: this is called the "dependent intestine sign". The pancreas is limited to cephalic portion (yellow dotted area).

The "dependent stomach sign" and "dependent intestine sign" (201) have been described as indirect radiological signs of the ADP. These are the presence of the stomach and/or some intestinal loops in the bed of the agennesic pancreas, next to the splenic vein (Figure 4-2). These signs are useful in differentiating the ADP from the fatty infiltration of the pancreas that is usually seen in pancreatic atrophy or in case of pancreatic lipomatosis (202). In addition, the "pseudo agenesis" of the pancreas that corresponds to the atrophy of the body and the tail of the pancreas (secondary to acute or chronic pancreatitis) may also mimic the ADP. In this case, the MRCP is crucial to differentiate the two entities: the dorsal duct of the pancreas is either absent or very short in the ADP whereas it should be entirely visualized in the "pseudo agenesis" of the pancreas (185).

It is worth noting that after pancreatic surgery (total or left pancreatectomy), the pancreatic bed would not contain any intestinal loops and therefore there will be neither "dependent intestinal sign" nor "dependent stomach sign" (203).

5. Treatment

Treatment should be tailored to the clinical characteristics of each patient:

For asymptomatic patients in whom ADP is discovered incidentally, regular monitoring of blood glucose levels and glycosylated hemoglobin (HbA1c) is necessary due to the High risk of diabetes (204).

Patients with diabetes need insulin therapy and those with exocrine insufficiency require pancreatic enzyme replacement therapy (204).

Endoscopic sphincterotomy with stenting of the main pancreatic has been seems an adequate and a reasonable therapeutic solution for patients with recurrent acute pancreatitis due to the ADP (205).

Patients with adenocarcinoma on residual pancreas should undergo a duodeno-pancreatectomy (whenever possible oncologically) however with endocrine and exocrine insufficiency as inevitable consequence (206).

CHAPTER 5

THE ANSA PANCREATICA

Ansa pancreatica is a very rare variation of pancreatic ducts' fusion in which the Santorini duct forms an inverted "S" and connects to a lateral branch of the main pancreatic duct (the Wirsung) (207).

According to a systematic review by Sotirios et al. in 2019 (208), the ansa pancreatica corresponds to the obliteration of the distal portion of the accessory pancreatic duct near its junction with the main pancreatic duct. The accessory duct is then replaced by a hook-shaped fine channel that serves as a communication between the dorsal and ventral ductal systems. This channel is formed by the proximal part of the accessory duct, the lower branch of the ventral duct and the lower branch of the dorsal duct (208, 209) (Figure 5-1). This channel ends at the level of the minor papilla which may be either permeable or obliterated.

Some hypotheses suggest that this ductal communication (ansa pancreatica) ensures a compensation of the obliteration either of the accessory duct or of the minor papilla. So, it would avoid any pancreatic drainage disturbance (208, 210).

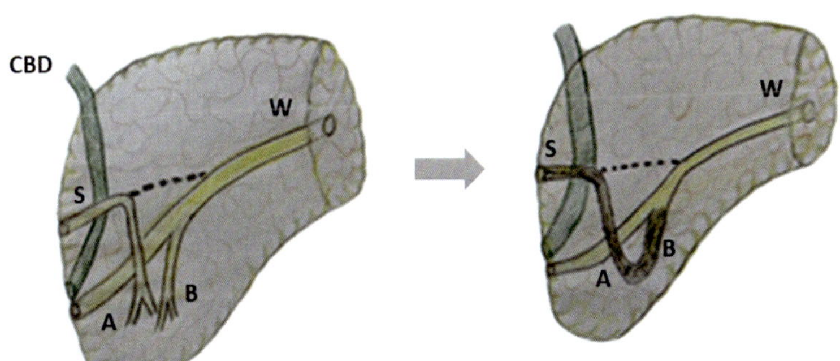

Figure 5-1: Ansa pancreatica formation. First, there is an obliteration (dotted line) of the accessory pancreatic duct (the Santorini) at its proximal side where it should normally join the main pancreatic duct (the Wirsung). Second, the ansa pancreatica is formed when the inferior branch (A) of the Santorini (S) joins the inferior branch (B) of the Wirsung (W).

Actually, 2 types of ansa pancreatica have been reported in the literature (figures 5-2 and 5-3) (211).

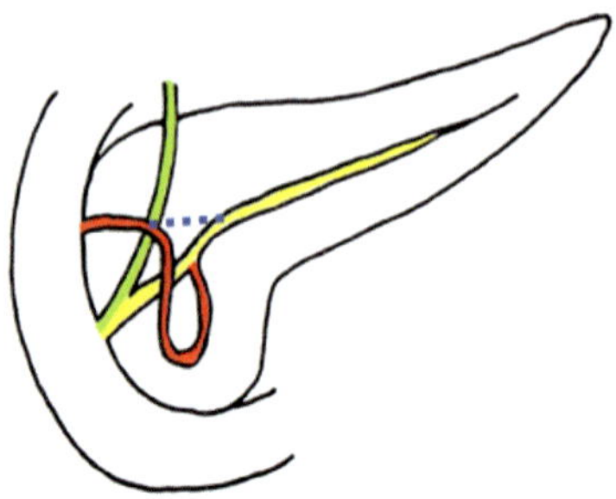

Figure 5-2: Ansa pancreatica type 1: Agenesis or obliteration (dotted line) of the proximal portion of the accessory pancreatic duct (the Santorini). The ansa pancreatic (red duct) is formed by the fusion of the inferior branches of the Santorini and the Wirsung (yellow duct). The latter ends in this case in the major papilla.

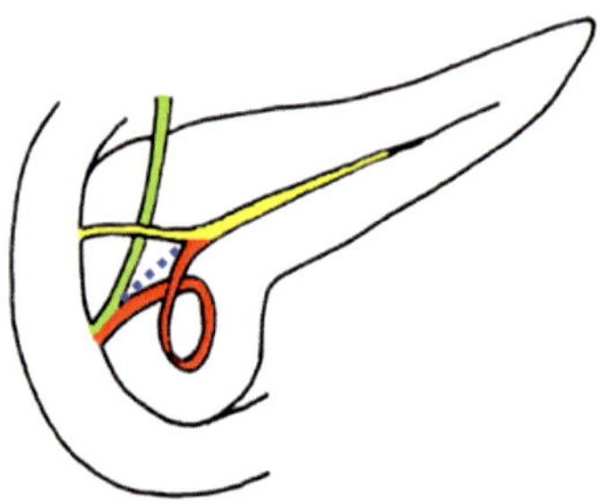

Figure 5-3: Ansa pancreatica type 2: Agenesis or obliteration of the proxiaml portin of the ventral duct (dotted line). The ansa pancreatica (red duct) is formed by the fusion of the inferior branches of the ventral and the dorsal pancreatic ducts. In this case, the main pancreatic duct (yellow duct) that corresponds to the dorsal duct in this case, ends into the minor papilla. In addition, the ansa pancreatica joins the main pancreatic duct at a variable distance from the minor papilla.

1. Epidemiology

The published studies about ansa pancreatica have been based either on anatomical-cadaveric examination or on ERCP and/or MRPC reports.

The ansa pancreatica was first described by Dawson and Langman in 1961 thanks to their anatomical and radiological study of cadaveric subjects (212). Their findings are as follows:

- This ductal anomaly was found in 17% of subjects.
- In 66% of cases, this duct was obliterated at its junction with the duodenum, despite a visible minor papilla.

Kamisawa et al. (213) reported in 1998 an endoscopic study showing a 13.6% incidence of ansa pancreatica in 213 patients presenting with biliopancreatic disease. The incidence of an impermeable minor papilla in these cases of ansa pancreatica was nearly 80%, which is noticeably higher than that reported by Dawson and Langman.

However, recent studies based either on MRCP or cadaveric examination, found a low incidence of ansa pancreatica (Table 5-1).

Table 5-1: Incidence of ansa pancreatica in the literature

Authors	Year	Country	NOP	Type of study	Incidence of AnP
Langman and Dawson (212)	1961	Canada	120	Cadaveric	17 %
Kamisawa et al. (213)	1998	Japan	213	Endoscopic (ERCP)	13.6 %
Liessi et al. (214)	2010	Italy	300	Radiological (S-MRCP)	1 %
Adibelli et al. (215)	2016	Turkey	1158	Radiological (MRCP)	1.2 %
Hayashi et al. (216)	2016	Japan	660	Radiological (MRCP)	1.2 %
Narayanan and Shabna (217)	2017	India	50	Cadaveric	2 %

AnP: Ansa Pancreatica; **NOP:** Number of Patients

Narayanan and Shabna reported in 2017 (217) a cadaveric study of the pancreatic ductal system in 50 subjects from an Indian population and found an incidence of 2% of ansa pancreatica. This low incidence, in contrast to that (17%) of the cadaveric study of Dawson and Langman (212), suggests a possible role of racial factors in the world distribution of ansa pancreatica.

The ansa pancreatica is actually considered as an adult condition. Indeed, only two cases of ansa pancreatica in child have been reported to date (218, 219).

2. Clinical Signs

The main clinical presentation of ansa pancreatica in symptomatic patients is acute pancreatitis. Indeed, several case reports of ansa pancreatica associated with necrotizing or interstitial edematous acute idiopathic pancreatitis (210, 220, 221).

According to Ishii et al. in 1998 (222), approximately 7% of patients with ansa pancreatica have at least one episode of acute pancreatitis.

In 2016, the first attempt to determine the exact unbiased incidence of ansa pancreatica and its correlation with acute pancreatitis was done by Hayashi et al. (216): they published a retrospective case-control study based on a Japanese population and the results were as follows:

- An incidence of 0.85% of ansa pancreatica in the control group.
- An incidence of 1.81% of ansa pancreatica in patients with a single episode of acute pancreatitis.
- An incidence of 11.1% of ansa pancreatica in patients with recurrent acute pancreatitis.
- The study also found that ansa pancreatica was more frequent in patients with alcoholic pancreatitis, but no exact and significant correlation could be obtained.

The study concluded that ansa pancreatica may be a predisposing factor for recurrent acute pancreatitis.

The pathophysiological involvement of the ansa pancreatica in the acute pancreatitis genesis remains however hypothetical and controversial. The suggested mechanism is that the ansa pancreatica ends in the main duct at an oblique angle, thus impeding the proper drainage of the pancreatic gland and causing acute pancreatitis. This is the same physio pathological explanation of acute pancreatitis related to sphincter of Oddi stenosis or to alcohol intoxication (223, 224).

Adibelli et al. published in 2016 (215) a radiological study (CPRM) of 1158 Turkish patients. They found that ansa pancreatica may be considered a chronic pancreatitis predisposing factor as the association between the two entities was statistically significant.

3. Imaging

The anatomical assessment of the pancreatic ducts may be done by either ERCP or MRCP. In addition, the latter, has the advantage of being a non-invasive imaging (225). However, ansa pancreatica is often described as a fine channel unlike in ERCP (Figure 5-4). This is probably due to the lack of injection of a radiopaque contrast medium that diffuses over higher intra-ductal pressures (226). On the other hand, the injection of secretin should increase the MRCP sensitivity in detecting pancreatic ductal variations, especially ansa pancreatica (208).

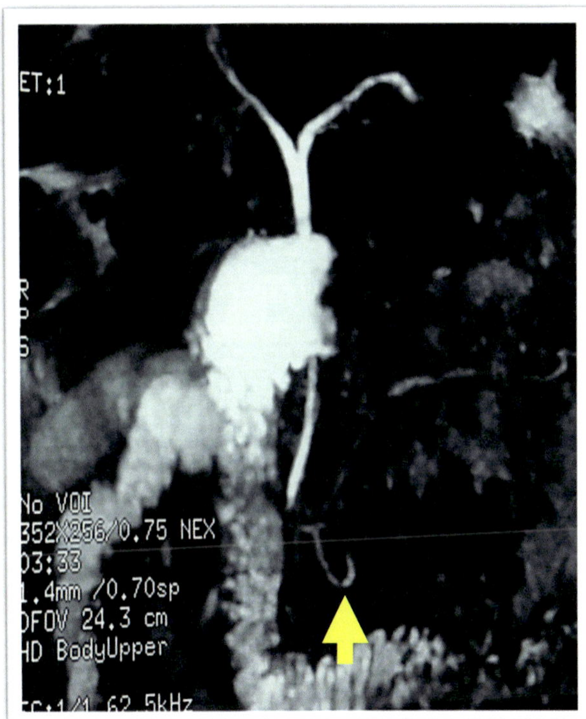

Figure 5-4: MRCP showing a looped pancreatic duct (yellow arrow) corresponding to an ansa pancreatica.

In addition, the diagnosis of ansa pancreatic may be done or confirmed with intra- or post-operative cholangiography if the patient undergoes a biliary surgery (227).

4. Treatment

Patients with ansa pancreatica shouldn't be treated unless they are symptomatic with recurrent or non-recurrent acute pancreatitis or with chronic pancreatitis.

There is no indication for laparoscopic cholecystectomy even though some authors may choose this option in case of idiopathic recurrent acute pancreatitis. Per or postoperative cholangiography could in this case reveal the ansa pancreatica (227).

4.1. Medical Treatment

Pancreatic enzymes replacement therapy (pancrelipase) is intended to slow down pancreatic excretion and to reduce intra-ductal pressure. Consequently, it would avoid acute or chronic pancreatitis (210).

4.2. Endoscopic Sphincterotomy of the Minor Papilla

The endoscopic sphincterotomy of the minor papilla seems to be a valid therapeutic option in both adults and children (218): it allows better functioning of the minor papilla and, above all, reduces pancreatic intra-ductal pressure. Moreover, the patients treated with endoscopic sphicterotomy of the minor papilla usually do not experience recurrence of acute pancreatitis.

Lopez-Duran et al. (228) described a technique using trans-gastric root (under endoscopic ultrasound control) to puncture the ansa pancreatica and to cannulate the accessory pancreatic duct. This allows to canulate the minor papilla so as it become easily detectable. The sphincterotomy of the minor papilla with this "Rendezvous" technique and pancreatic stenting should then be performed to ensure adequate pancreatic drainage. This would obviously prevent acute pancreatitis flare-ups (Figure 5-5).

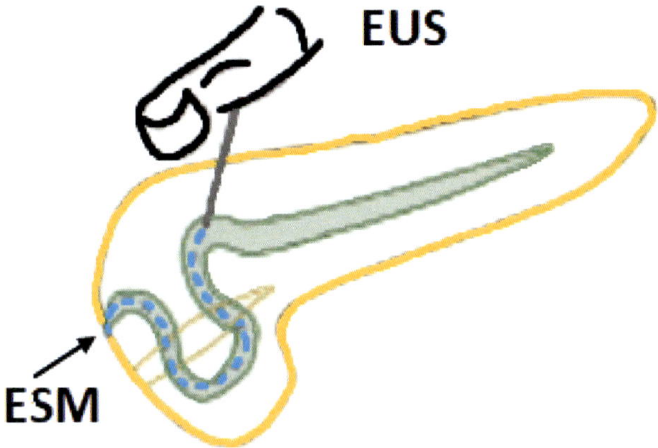

Figure 5-5: Rendezvous technique: endoscopic ultrasound (EUS) guided puncture of the pancreatic duct with endoscopic cannulation and sphincterotomy of the minor papilla (ESM).

CHAPTER 6

CONCLUSION

Congenital anomalies of the pancreas and pancreatic ducts are uncommon and mostly asymptomatic. These anomalies are pancreas divisum, annular pancreas, agenesis of the dorsal pancreas and ansa pancratica. The pancreas divisum is the most common malformation.

These congenital entities are usually incidentally discovered in asymptomatic patients. However, they may be undetected, in which case they would cause recurrent acute pancreatitis and even chronic pancreatitis.

The development of imaging techniques in recent decades has made it possible to better study these malformations, but their management remains difficult and, above all, not consensual.

The incidence of pancreas divisum is around 10% of the general population. It results from the defect in the fusion of the ductal systems of the dorsal and the ventral pancreatic embryonic remnants during the 7th week of embryonic life. The result is a ventral pancreatic duct that drains through the major papilla and a dominant dorsal pancreatic duct that drains most of the gland through the minor papilla which is not always properly functional (variable patency between patients).

More than 95% of patients with pancreas divisum are asymptomatic, and the anomaly is usually discovered fortuitously on abdominal imaging (CT-scan, CPRM) performed for other symptoms or indications.

The etiopathogenic role of pancreas divisum in pancreatic disease has been suggested regarding first its high incidence in idiopathic recurrent acute pancreatitis and second the favorable outcomes of treatment options targeting the minor papilla. However, the definitive incrimination of pancreas divisum in pancreatic disease is still a matter of debate because actually there is no well-identified and established evidence of causality. On the other hand, it has been suggested that pancreas divisum predisposes to pancreatic disease in association with other conditions such as genetic mutations.

The S-CPRM is currently the reference imaging for the diagnosis of pancreas divisum. Nevertheless, no investigations should be considered or recommended for patients with asymptomatic pancreas divisum.

For patients with recurrent acute pancreatitis, endoscopic sphincterotomy of the minor papilla currently remains the first-line treatment. Minor papilla surgery has comparable results but it must be reserved for patients in whom endoscopic sphincterotomy has failed. The outcome of endoscopic or surgical treatment is variable with maximum benefit in patients with recurrent acute pancreatitis. The outcome is poorer in patients with chronic pancreatitis, and it is the poorest in patients with chronic abdominal pain.

For patients with pancreas divisum and chronic pancreatitis, surgical treatment should be considered after failure of at least one attempt of endoscopic sphincterotomy of the minor papilla. In this case, therapeutic objective should be symptom control with several options such as resting the gland by jejunal feeding or somatostatin analogues and celiac plexus blockade. Other surgical options such as the latero-lateral pancreaticojejunal anastomosis (Frey or Puestow procedure) and the new technique of total pancreatectomy with pancreatic islet auto transplantation may be conceivable in some patients.

The annular pancreas is usually diagnosed in the neonatal period as a surgical emergency because of duodenal obstruction. In this case a diamond-shaped duodeno-duodenal anastomosis is recommended. Adult patients with annular pancreas are usually asymptomatic and do not require any therapeutic management. Although surgery remains the mainstay of treatment in patients with duodenal obstruction, the majority of symptomatic adults, including those with acute recurrent pancreatitis, require no further invasive treatment.

The dorsal agenesis of the pancreas is an extremely rare congenital anomaly, which results from the embryological failure of the dorsal pancreatic bud to form the body and tail of the pancreas. The clinical presentation of the ADP is highly variable. In general, it is incidentally discovered in asymptomatic patients, otherwise abdominal pain, diabetes and recurrent acute pancreatitis are the most common clinical manifestations. However, it is worth noting that annular pancreas may be associated with cystic lesions of the residual pancreas or with bilio-pancreatic neoplasms such as IPMN of the pancreas and ampullary adenocarcinomas.

Annular pancreas with diabetes should be managed with insulin therapy whereas endoscopic sphincterotomy is indicated in the case of recurrent acute pancreatitis, unless there is an associated tumor pathology.

Finally, the ansa pancreatica is a very rare congenital anomaly of the pancreatic ducts related to an embryological fusion defect of the pancreatic ducts, resulting in a very thin, inverted "S" shaped or loop shaped ductal communication between the Santorini and the Wirsung. This is a predisposing condition for recurrent acute pancreatitis.

Among the therapeutic options, endoscopic sphincterotomy of the minor papilla seems to be a valid option for the treatment of symptomatic adults or even children with ansa pancreatica. It would ensure a better functioning of the minor papilla and would decrease considerably the pancreatic intra-ductal pressure.

In conclusion, congenital pancreatic anomalies are uncommon and usually asymptomatic. However, symptomatic patients present mainly with recurrent acute pancreatitis with possible progression to chronic pancreatitis or degeneration. In addition, the physician should look for other etiopathogenic factors of acute pancreatitis such as dyslipidemia, drugs, autoimmune pancreatitis, and associated bilio-pancreatic congenital anomaly (e.g., association of a PDiv with an annular pancreas).

It is worth noting that the pancreatic ductal anomalies have benefited greatly from advances not only in imaging techniques (especially since the advent of MRCP and ERCP), but also in surgical and endoscopic techniques.

The main therapeutic objective of a congenital pancreatic anomaly is to relieve pancreatic intraductal pressure. That is why the endoscopic sphincterotomy of the minor papilla is currently the treatment of choice in symptomatic patients. A medical treatment aiming to inhibit pancreatic secretions (with pancreatic enzymes replacement therapy) may also be attempted. And finally, surgery remains the last resort therapeutic option and must be discussed on a case-by-case basis.

REFERENCES

Part 1: Cystic dilatation of bile ducts

1. George N Baison, Morgan M Bonds, William S Helton, Richard A Kozarek. Choledochal cysts: Similarities and differences between Asian and Western countries. World J Gastroenterol. 2019 Jul: 25(26): 3334-43.
2. Liu Y, Sun J, Guo S, Liu Z, Zhu M, Zhang Z. The distal classification and management of choledochal cyst in adults: Based on the relation between cyst and pancreatic duct. JAMA Int Med. 2017 Feb: 96(12): 1-5.
3. Budipramana VS, Saraswati PA. Type VI choledochal cyst: A case report. Int J Surg. 2020 Feb; 68(1): 11-4.
4. Yoshinori Hamada, Hisami Ando, Terumi Kamisawa, Takao Itoi, Naoto Urushihara, Tsugumichi Koshinaga, Takeshi Saito, Hideki Fujii, Yoshiki Morotomi. Diagnostic criteria for congenital biliary dilatation 2015. J Hepatobiliary Pancreat 2016; 23(2): 342–346.
5. Weng R, Hu W, Cai S, Guo X, Luo Q. Prenatal diagnosis and prognosis assessment of congenital choledochal cyst in 21 cases. J Obstet Gynaecol. 2016 Apr; 36(3): 324-7.
6. Ragot E, Mabrut J-Y, Ouaïssi M, Sauvanet A, Dokmak S, et al. Pancreaticobiliary Maljunctions in European Patients with Bile Duct Cysts: Results of the Multicenter Study of the French Surgical Association (AFC). World J Surg. 2017 Feb; 41(2): 538-45.
7. de Albuquerque VVML, De Macedo FP, Costa KG, Rodrigues Seixas Nunes Z, da Silva Junior RA. Choledochal cyst-unusual presentation in the adult phase: case report. Int J Surg Res. 2020 Apr; 51(2): 33-6.
8. Florian Friedmacher. Kathryn E. Ford. Mark Davenport. Choledochal malformations: global research, scientific advances and key controversies. Pediatr Surg Int. 2018 Oct; 5(1): 1-9.
9. Mohamed I. Kassem, Hany M. El-Haddad, Mohamed T. Elriwini. Surgical outcome of choledochal cysts in adults: a prospective cohort study. Egypt J Surg. 2017; 36(1): 274-82.
10. Robert E, Gross. Idiopathic dilatation of the common bile duct in children. J Pediatr. 1933 Nov; 3(5); 730-755.

11. Friedmacher F, Ford KE, Davenport M. Choledochal malformations: global research, scientific advances and key controversies. Pediatr Surg Int. 2019 Mar; 35(3): 273-82.
12. Fatih Altıntoprak, Mustafa Yener Uzunoğlu, Enis Dikicier, and İsmail Zengin. Choledochal cysts-Classification, physiopathology, and clinical course. Integr Cancer Ther. 2016 Oct; 3(5): 588-592.
13. Sen SS, Menon P, Solanki S, Bhatia A, Sen IM. Acute pancreatitis with Cullen's sign presentation in a case of mixed type I and II choledochal cyst. J of Pediatric Surg. 2019 Oct; 54(10): 2187-90.
14. Xia H-T, Wang J, Yang T, Liang B, Zeng J-P, Dong J-H. Sphincter of Oddi Dysfunction and the Formation of Adult Choledochal Cyst Following Cholecystectomy: A Retrospective Cohort Study. Medicine. 2015 Nov; 94(47): 2088.
15. Boussouni K, Taam I, Dafiri R. Dilatation kystique du canal cystique chez un nouveau né de 20 jours : à propos d'un cas. J Afr Hepato Gastroenterol. 2016 Oct; 10(3): 151-4.
16. Soares KC, Goldstein SD, Ghaseb MA, Kamel I, Hackam DJ, Pawlik TM. Pediatric choledochal cysts: diagnosis and current management. Pediatr Surg Int. 2017 Jan; 33(6): 637-50.
17. Sastry AV, Abbadessa B, Wayne MG, et al. What is the incidence of biliary carcinoma in choledochal cysts, when do they develop, and how should it affect management? World J Surg. 2015; 39(1): 487–492.
18. Tahara K, Ishimaru Y, Fujino J, Suzuki M, Hatanaka M, Igarashi A. Association of extrahepatic bile duct duplication with pancreaticobiliary maljunction and congenital biliary dilatation in children: A case report and literature review. Surg Today. 2013; 43(7): 800 – 5.
19. Miyano T, Yamataka A, Kato Y, Sagawa O, Lane G, Takamizawa S et al. Hepaticoenterostomy after excision of choledochal cyst in children: a 30-year experience with 180 cases. J Pediatr Surg. 1996; 31: 1417-21.
20. Manavi, E. Stavride, M. Theodorou, M. Kosmidou, A. Theodorakopoulos, Thessaloniki GR, Thessaloniki, Thessaloniki GR. Choledochal cysts: lesions to follow or to ignore. Eur Radiol. 2019; 1:(1)14.
21. Kim SH, Lim JH, Yoon HK, et al. Choledochal cyst: comparison of MR and conventional cholangiography. Clin Radiol. 2000; 55: 378-83.
22. Fan F, Xu D-P, Xiong Z-X, Li H-J, Xin H-B, Zhao H, et al. Clinical significance of intrapancreatic choledochal cyst excision in surgical

management of type I choledochal cyst. J Int Med Res. 2018 Mar; 46(3): 1221-9.
23. Tannuri ACA, Hara LA d'A, Paganoti G de F, Andrade W de C, Tannuri U. Choledochal cysts in children: How to Diagnose and Operate on. Clinics. 2020; 75(2): 1539.
24. Nabil Boudjenan Serradj1, Benali Tabeti1, Anisse Tidjane1, Noureddine Benmaarouf1. Le cholédococèle: une variété rare de dilatation kystique congénitale des voies biliaires. Pan African Medical J. 2018 Mar; 29(2): 156: 4.
25. Hamada, Terumi Kamisawa, Hideki Fujii, Tsugumichi Koshinaga, Yoshiki Morotomi Takeshi Saito, Takao Itoi, Kenitiro Kaneko, Hiroaki Fukuzawa, Hisami Ando. Classification of pancreaticobiliary maljunction and clinical features inchildren. J Hepatobiliary Pancreat Sci 2017 Jul; 24(1); 449-455.
26. Jihane Rizkou, Khadija Krati, Safa Raoudi, Chama Elmnjra, Adil Ait Errami, Safia Obaha, Zouhour Samlani. Caroli Syndrome: about a case Report and Revew of litterature. Sch J Med Case Rep. 2020 Nov; 8(11); 941-944.
27. Banks JS, Saigal G, D'Alonzo JM, Bastos MD, Nguyen NV. Choledochal Malformations: Surgical Implications of Radiologic Findings. Am J Roentgen. 2018 Avr; 210(4): 748-60.
28. Machado NO, Chopra PJ, Al-Zadjali A, Younas S. Choledochal Cyst in Adults: Etiopathogenesis, Presentation, Management, and Outcome—Case Series and Review.Gastroenterol Res Prac. 2015 Jul; 2015(3): 1-10.
29. Huang CT, Lee HC, Chen WT, et al. Usefulness of magnetic resonance cholangiopancreatography in pancreatobiliary abnormalities in pediatric patients. Pediatr Neonatol. 2011;(52): 332-6.
30. Ahmed Azahouani1, Najlae Zaari1, Fatine El Aissaoui1, Mohamed Hida1, Mohamed Fitri1, Larbi Benradi1, Houssain Benhaddou1. Kyste du cholédoque rompu: revue de la littérature Cyst of the broken common bile duct: literature review. Pan Afr med J. 2019 Jul; 33 (2); 33-276.
31. Goldman M, Pranikoff T. Biliary Disease in Children. Curr Gastroenterol Rep. 2011 Avr; 13(2): 193-201.
32. Badebarin D, Aslanabadi S, Teimouri-Dereshki A, Jamshidi M, Tarverdizadeh T, Shad K, et al. Different clinical presentations of choledochal cyst among infants and older children: A 10-year retrospective study. Medicine. 2017 Avr; 96(17): 6679.

33. Ronnekleiv-Kelly SM, Soares KC, Ejaz A, Pawlik TM. Management of choledochal cysts: Curr Opin Gastroenterol.2016 Ma 32 (3); 225-31.
34. Ghizlane Erraoui. 2018. Dilatation kystique congénitale du cholédoque à propos de 09 cas. Doctoral thesis [236], Medecine School of Marakch Morocco. 63-64.
35. Ahmed Azahouani1, Najlae Zaari1, Fatine El Aissaoui, Mohamed Hida, Mohamed Fitri, Larbi Benradi, Houssain Benhaddou. Kyste du cholédoque rompu: revue de la littérature. Pan Afr Med J. 2019 Jul; 33(2) 276.
36. Norman Oneil Machado, Pradeep J. Chopra, Adil Al-Zadjali, and Shahzad Younas. Choledochal Cyst in Adults: Etiopathogenesis, Presentation, Management, and Outcome—Case Series and Review. Gastroent Res Pract. 2015 Jul; 2015(3) 1-10.
37. Karolin Baumgartner, Jens Kübler, Michael Bitzer, Hans Bösmüller, Marius Horger. Caroli's syndrome. Rofo. 2020 Feb; 192(2): 119-122.
38. Ishibashi H, Shimada M, Kamisawa T, Fujii H, Hamada Y, Kubota M, et al. Japanese clinical practice guidelines for congenital biliary dilatation. J Hepatobiliary Pancreat Sci. 2017 Jan; 24(1): 1–16.
39. Lane E, Murray k. Neonatal Cholestasis. Pediatr Clin N Am. 2017; 64(3): 621–639.
40. Yuxin He, Zhuwen Yu and Weichang Chen.Type IV choledochal cyst with polycystickidney disease: a case report.BMC Gastroenterol. 2020 Sep; 20(306); 1-5.
41. Oshua Q. Knowlton and Lisa H. Lowe. Congenital Hepatobiliary Anomalies. Radio Key. 2015 Dec; 2(1); 38.
42. Subramony R, Kittisarapong N, Barata I, Nelson M. Choledochal Cyst Mimicking Gallbladder with Stones in à Six-Year-Old with Right-sided Abdominal Pain.West J Emerg Med. 2015 Jul; 16(4); 568-71.
43. Kuntharee Traisrisilp. Fuanglada Tongprasert. Komson Wannasai. Theera Tongsong MD. Giant choledochal cyst and infantile polycystic kidneys as prenatal sonographic features of Caroli syndrome. J Clin Ultrasound.2019 Jul; 1(3): 1-4.
44. James S. Banks, Gaurav Saigal, Joseph M. D'Alonzo, Maria D'Almeida B astos, Nguyen V. Nguyen. Choledochal Malformations: Surgical Implications of Radiologic Findings. AJR Am J Roentgenol. 2018 Apr; 210(4): 748-760.
45. Venkata Vishwanath Reddych, Ashok Kumar, Manas Aggarwal, Kailash Chand Kurdia. Type VI choledochal cyst with gall bladder carcinoma. J Gastrointest Surg. 2019 Dec 29; 12(12): 232715.

46. Santiago, Rui Loureiro, Luis Curvo-Semedo, Cristina Marques. Congenital Cystic Lesions of the Biliary Tree. AJR Am J Roentgenol. 2012 Apr; 198 (4): 825-35.
47. S. Mannai, T. Kraiem, N.Gharbi, L. Haoues, H. Mestiri, M, T, Khalfallah. La dilatation kystique congénitale du cholédoque. Ann Chir. 2006; 2(1): 369-74.
48. Dry Ferdaous. 2014. Dilatation Kystique Congénitale Du Cholèdoque à propos 09 cas, Dcotoral thesis [66]. Medical school of Fes, Morocco. 88-89.
49. Fanny Yeung, Adrian C H Fung, Patrick H. Y. Chung Kenneth K. Y Wong. Short-term and long-term outcomes after Roux-en-Y hepaticojejunostomy versus hepaticoduodenostomy following laparoscopic excision of choledochal cyst in children. Surg Endosc. 2019 Jul; 34(5); 2172-2177.
50. 95 Travis Ackermann, Fracs Dean Spilias. Type VI choledochal cyst: a rare entity. ANZ J Surg. 2020 May; 1(3); 1-2.
51. Amarjothi JMV, Ramasamy V, Jesudasan J, NaganathBabu OL. Type VI Choledochal Cysts-Case Report and Review of Literature. Surg J (NY). 2019 Aug 23; 5(3):e82-e86. doi: 10.1055/s-0039-1693652.
52. Visser BC, Suh I, Way LW, Kang SM. Congenital choledochal cysts in adults. Arch Surg 1960; 2004; 139: 855–860; discussion, 860–862.
53. Lilly JR. The surgical treatment of choledochal cyst. Surg. Gynecol Obstet 1979; 149: 36-42.
54. Kaneyama K, Yamataka A, Kobayashi H, Lane GJ, Miyano T. Mixed type I and II choledochal cyst: A new clinical subtype? Pediatr Surg Int. 2005; 21(2): 911-3.
55. Rania Kronfli, Mark Davenport. Insights into the pathophysiology and classification of type choledochal malformation. J Pediatr Surg. 2020 May; 2(1); 1-5.
56. Hamada, Terumi Kamisawa, Hideki Fujii, Tsugumichi Koshinaga, Yoshiki Morotomi, Takeshi Saito, Takao Itoi, Kenitiro Kaneko, Hiroaki Fukuzawa, Hisami Ando.Classification of pancreaticobiliary maljunction and clinical features in children. J Hepatobiliary Pancreat Sci. 2017 Aug; 24(8): 449-455.
57. Bertrand Le Roy, Johan Gagniere, Laura Filaire, Mikael Fontarensky, Constance Hordonneau, Emmanuel Buc. Pancreaticobiliary maljunction and choledochal cysts: from embryogenesis to therapeutics aspects. Surg Radiol Anat. 2016 Mar; 38(2); 1053–1060.
58. Taqi Toufeeq Khan, Nadeem Ahmad.Pancreaticobiliary Maljunctions in European Patients with Bile Duct Cysts.World J Surg. 2018 Nov; 42(11): 3817-3818.

59. Maryam Abbaoui. Dilatation kystique du cholédoque à prorps 07 cas, [Thèse 364], Médecine Rabat, 2019, 119-120.
60. Funabiki T, Matsubara T, Ochia LM, watanabe Y, Seo T, Harada T, et al. Biliary carcinogenesis in pancreaticobiliary maljunction. J Hepatobil Pancreat Surg. 1997; 4(3): 405-11.
61. Janakie Surgham, Eric M, Yoshida, Charles H, Scudamore. Choledochal cysts.Part 1 of 3: Classification and pathogenesis. J Can Chir. 2009 Oct ; 52(5); 434-40.
62. Kamisawa T, Kaneko K, Itoi T, Ando H. Pancreaticobiliary maljunction and congenital biliary dilatation. Lancet Gastroenterol Hepatol. 2017 Aug; 2(8): 610-8.
63. Sindhura Kollia Simcha Weissmanb Emmanuel Oforic Khoi Paul Dang-Hoa Praneeth Bandarua, Kruthika Bachalia, Evangelos Tsipotisc, Denzil Etiennec, Madhavi Reddy, Abraham Jelinc, Krishna Gurram. Minor Papillary Relief in a Type IA Choledochal Cyst: A Case Report andReview of the Literature.Case Rep Gastroenterol. 2020 Apr; 14(2): 116–123.
64. Terumi Kamisawa, Hisami Ando, Masafumi Suyama, Mitsuo Shimada, Yuji Morine, Hiroshi Shimada. Japanese clinical practice guidelines for pancreaticobiliary maljunction. J Gastroenterol 2012 Jul; 47(3); 731–759.
65. Nakamura, Tatsuma Sakaguchi, Hiroaki Yanagimoto, Kentaro Inoue, Masanori Kon. Duodenogastric regurgitation in hepaticoduodenostomy after excision ofcongenital biliary dilatation (choledochal cyst). J Pediatr Surg. 2017 Oct; 52 (10); 1621-1624.
66. Jesus Morales-Maza, Jorge Humberto Rodríguez-Quintero, Sonia Cortés-Vázquez, Luis Cruz-Benítez. Giant choledochal cyst presenting during third trimester of pregnancy. BMJ Case Rep. 2018 Ju; 13(2); 1-4.
67. Sarin YK, Sengar M, Puri AS. Forme fruste choledochal cyst. Indian Pediatr. 2005 Nov; 42(11): 1153-5.
68. Ayako Ono, Shigeki Arizono, Hiroyoshi Isoda, Kaori Togashi, Imaging of Pancreaticobiliary Maljunction. Radio Graphics. 2020 Apr; 40(2); 1-15
69. Michaelides M, Dimarelos V, Kostantinou D, Bintoudi A, Tzikos F, Kyriakou V, Rodokalakis G, Tsitouridis I. A new variant of Todani type I choledochal cyst. Imaging evaluation. Hyppokratia 2011 Apr; 15(2); 174-177.
70. Honnavara Srinivasan P, Anbalagan A, Shanmugasundaram R, Obla Lakshmanamoorthy N. Management of Choledochal Cysts at a

Tertiary Care Centre: A Nine-Year Experience from India.Surg Res Pract. 2020 Avr; 2020(2); 1-8.
71. Kenny T. Quang, Justin L. Hunter, John W. Wilson, and Jon D. Simmons. Choledochal Cyst Originating From the Cystic Duct. Am Surg. 2020 Sep; 3(5); 1-2.
72. Salma Foura. Les dilatations kystiques congénitales de la voie biliaire principale chez l'enfant, [Thèse 036], Médecine Marrakch, 2017, 89-90.
73. Sean M. Ronnekleiv-Kelly, Kevin C-Soares, Aslam Ejaz, and Timothy M. Pawlik. Management of choledochal cysts. Curr Opin Gastroenterol. 2016; 32(2): 1-7.
74. Angela J. Marolf. Diagnostic Imaging of the Hepatobiliary System. Vet Clin North Am Small Anim Pract. 2017 Ma; 47(3): 555-68.
75. Paris C, Bejjani J, Beaunoyer M, Ouimet A. Endoscopic retrograde cholangiopancreatography is useful and safe in children. J Pediatr Surg. 2010; 45(2); 938-42.
76. E Frampas, Moussaly, H Eloury, JC, LE Neel, et B Dupas. Cholangio-pancreatographie par IRM des kystes du cholédoque. J Radiol. 1999; 80(1): 1659-63.
77. Otto AK, Neal MD, Slivka AN, Kane TD. An appraisal of endoscopic retrograde cholangiopancreatography for pancreaticobiliary disease in children: our institutional experience in 231 cases. Surg Endosc. 2011; 25(2): 2536-40.
78. Saito T, Terui K, Mitsunaga T, Nakata M, Yoshida H. Significance of imaging modalities for preoperative evaluation of the pancreaticobiliary system in surgery for pediatric choledochal Cyst. J Hepatobiliary Pancreat Sci. 2016 Ju; 23(6): 347-52.
79. Rajnish A, Gambhir S, Das BK, Saxena R. Classifying choledochal cysts using hepatobiliary scintigraphy. Clin Nucl Med. 2000; 25: 996-9.
80. Myung-Joon Kim, Seok Joo Han, Choon Sik Yoon, Joo Hee Kim, Jung-Tak Oh, Ki Sup Chung, Hyung Sik Yoo. Using MR Cholangiopancreatography to Reveal Anomalous Pancreaticobiliary Ductal Union in Infants and Children with Choledochal Cysts. Am J Roentgenol. 2002 Jul; 3(2); 209-214.
81. Maria Hendrina Antoinette van den Eijnden Ruben H. de Kleine Henkjan J. Verkade Jim C. H. Wilde, Paul M. J. G. Peeters Jan B. F. Hulscher. Controversies in Choledochal Malformations: A Survey among Dutch Pediatric Surgeons. Eur J Pediatr Surg. oct 2015; 25(2).
82. Sugandhi N, Agarwala S, Bhatnagar V, Singh MK, Sharma R. Liver histology in choledochal cyst- pathological changes and response to

surgery: the overlooked aspect? Pediatr Surg Int. 2014; 30(2): 205–211.
83. Takahashi T, Shimotakahara A, Okazaki T, et al. Intraoperative endoscopy during choledochal cyst excision: extended long-term follow-up compared with recent cases. J Pediatr Surg. 2010; 45(2): 379–382.
84. Çamlıdağ İ, Nural MS, Danacı M, Karabıçak İ, Karabulut K. Cholangiocarcinoma Arising from a Type VI Biliary Cyst: A Case Report and Review of the Literature. J Radiol Case Rep. Oct 2015; 2015(2): 1-4.
85. Mutignani, M., Tringali, A., Costamagna, G. Therapeutic Biliary Endoscopy. Endoscop. 2004; 36(2): 147-59.
86. Vijayaraghavan P, Lal R, Sikora SS, Poddar U, Yachha SK. Experience with choledochal cysts in infants. Pediatr Surg Int. 2006; 22(10): 803-7.
87. Karim A. Caroli's disease. Indian Pediatr. 2004; 41(1): 848-50.
88. Abdulrahman Alabdulkareem a, Tameem Almahmoud a, Husam Al-Tahan a, Sundas Javad b, Maher Al Hatlani c. Etiology and clinical characteristics of pediatric acute pancreatitis in Saudi Arabia: a 20-year experience from a single tertiary center. Int J Pediatr Adolesc Med. 2018 Jan; 5(1): 13-7.
89. Jun Fujishiro, Kouji Masumoto, Yasuhisa Urita, Toko Shinkai, Chikashi Gotoh. Pancreatic complications in pediatric choledochal cysts. J Pediatr Surg. 2013Jan; 48(9): 1897–1902.
90. Akisik MF, Sandrasegaran K, Aisen AA, Maglinte DD, Sherman S, Lehman GA. Dynamicsecretin-enhanced MR cholangio-pancreatography. Radio Graphics. 2006 Ma; 26(3): 665-77.
91. Mei Diao, Long Li, and Wei Cheng. Timing of Choledochal Cyst Perforation. Hepatology. 2020 Feb; 71(2); 753-756.
92. Benchellal ZA, Simon E, d'Alte´roche L, et al. Choledochal cyst rupture during pregnancy. Gastroenterol Clin Biol. 2009; 33(2): 390-1.
93. Vanessa A. Lewis, Sharon Z. Adam, Paul Nikolaidis, Cecil Wood, James G. Wu, Vahid Yaghmai, Frank H. Miller.Imaging of choledochal cysts. Abdom Imaging 2015 Feb; 1(2) ; 1-14.
94. Ayako Ono, Shigeki Arizono, Hiroyoshi Isoda, Kaori Togashi. Imaging of Pancreaticobiliary Maljunction. Radiographics. 2020 Apr; 40 (2): 378-392.
95. Lawrence Ku, Marco A. Paez, Michael P. O'Leary, MD, Danielle M. Hari, FACS, Sofiya Reicher, Lawrence Ku, Marco A. Paez, Michael P. O'Leary, MD, Danielle M. Hari Facs. Type VI choledochal cyst

diagnosed on ERCP with direct cholangioscopy. Am S Gastroent Endoscop. 2019 Oct; 4(2): 458-460.

96. Kyuwhan Jung, Ho-Seong Han, PhD, Jai Young Cho, Yoo-Seok Yoon, Dae-Wook Hwang. Is Preoperative Subclassification of Type I Choledochal Cyst Necessary? Korean J Radiol. 2012 Feb; 13(1): 112-116.
97. Myung-Joon Kim, Seok Joo Han, Choon Sik Yoon, Joo Hee Kim, Jung-Tak Oh, Ki Sup Chung, Hyung Sik Yoo. Using MR Cholangiopancreatography to Reveal Anomalous Pancreaticobiliary Ductal Union in Infants and Children with Choledochal Cysts. Am J Roentgenol. 2002 Jul; 3(2); 209-214.
98. Kenny T. Quang, Justin L. Hunter, John W. Wilson, and Jon D. Simmons. Choledochal Cyst Originating From the Cystic Duct. Am Surg. 2020 Sep; 1(1); 1-1.
99. Judah JR, Draganov P V. Endoscopic therapy of benign biliary strictures. World Journal of Gastroenterology. World J Pediatr. 2007; 13(7): 3531 – 9.
100. Qianqian Wang, Suk Bae Moon, Jingyu Zang, Jun Liu, Jie Chen. Usefulness of pre-operative endoscopic retrograde cholangiopancreatography in diagnosis and management of forme fruste choledochal cyst in children. ANZ J Surg. 2020 Jun; 90(6): 1041-1045.
101. Anchu Rajnish, Sanjay Guimbhir, Berindra and Rajan Saxena. Classifying Choledochal Cysts Using Hepatobiliary Scintigraphy. Clin Nucl Med. 2000 Dec; 25(12): 996-9.
102. Emily Tommolino, Michael H Piper. Choledochal Cysts: Treatment and Management. Am J Gastroenterol. 2019 Ju; 5(1): 1-8.
103. Leila B.F, Asmae B.A, Anis Aski, Lasaad.D, Lotfi.H. Drainage biliaire percutané: efficacité et complications à court et à moyen terme à travers une série de 50 cas. Tunis Med. 2009; 87(1): 50-4.
104. Fujishiro J, Masumoto K, Urita Y, Shinkai T, Gotoh C. Pancreatic complications in pediatric choledochal cysts. J Pediatr Surg. 2013; 48(9): 1897–902.
105. Bhavsar MS, Vora HB, Giriyappa VH. Choledochal cysts: a review of literature. Saudi J Gastroenterol. 2012 Jul; 18(4): 230 – 6.
106. Bricha M, Dafiri R. Une cause inhabituelle d'un abdomen aigu chez l'enfant: La rupture spontanée d'un kyste du cholédoque. J Radio. 2007; 88(51): 692–3.
107. Linlin Zhu, Jing Xiong, Zhibao Lv, Jiangbin Liu, Xiong Huang and Weijue Xu. Type C Pancreaticobiliary Maljunction Is Associated With Perforated Choledochal Cyst in Children. Front Pediatr. 2020

With Perforated Choledochal Cyst in Children. Front Pediatr. 2020 Avr; 8(3): 1-6.
108. Marta Garzón-Benavides, Andrea Núñez-Ortiz, Teófilo López-Ruiz, Carmen Cepeda-Franco and Lourdes Gómez-Izquierdo. Pancreatobiliary maljunction: association with gallbladder cancer. Rev Esp Enferm Dig. 2019 Mar; 111(7); 568-570.
109. Omid Madadi-Sanjani Thomas C. Wirth Joachim F. Kuebler Claus Petersen Benno M. Ure. Choledochal Cyst and Malignancy: A Plea for Lifelong Follow-Up. Eur J Pediatr Surg. 2017 Nov; 4(1): 1-7.
110. Sindhura Kolli. Simcha Weissman, Emmanuel Ofori, Khoi Paul Dang-Ho, Praneeth Bandaru, Kruthika Bachali, Krishna Gurram. Minor Papillary Relief in a Type IA Choledochal Cyst: A Case Report and review of the Literature. Case Rep Gastroenterol. 2020 Jan; 14(1): 116–123.
111. Qing-Yu Liu, Dong-Ming Lai, Ming Gao, Yun-Le Wan, Xiao-Feng Lin, Hai-Gang Li, Bi-Ling Liang. MRI manifestations of adult choledochal cysts associated with biliary malignancy: a report of ten cases. Abdom Imaging. 2012 Jul; 38(5): 1061-70.
112. Mei Diao, Long Li, and Wei Cheng. Timing of Choledochal Cyst Perforation. Hepatology. 2020 Feb; 71(2): 753-756.
113. Uno K, TsushidaY, Kawasaki H, Ohmiya H. Development of intrahepatic cholelithiasis long after primary excision of choledochal cyst. J Am Coll Surg. 1996; 183(3); 45-48.
114. Jiachen Zheng, Zihanli, Yonqin Ye and Bin Wang. Short-Term Comlications After Laparoscopie Choledochal Cyst: Radical Surgery: Prevention and treatment. Front surg, 2020 Oct; 7(2); 1-5.
115. Ersin Gündoğan, Fatih Sümer, Muhammed Kadri Çolakoğlu, Egemen Çiçek, Cihan Gökler, Mehmet Can Aydın, Cüneyt Kayaalp. Laparoscopic resection of choledochal cysts in adults: a series from Turkey. Turk J Surg. 2019; 35 (3): 223-226.
116. Saalim Nazki, Ravi Prakash Kanojia, Monika Bawa, Vineet Binu, Sadhna Lal, Ashwani Sood, Ram Samujh. Robotic Excision of Choledochal Cyst with Hepaticoduodenostomy (HD): Report of HD Technique, Initial Experience, and Early Outcome. Eur J Pediater Surg. 2020 Jul; 2(1); 1-6.
117. Shui-qing Chi, Guo-qing Cao, Shuai Li, Jia-ling Guo, Xi Zhang, Ying Zhou, Shao-tao Tang. Outcomes in robotic versus laparoscopic-assisted choledochal cyst excision and hepaticojejunostomy in children. Surg Endosc. 2019 Nov; 29(11); 1486-1491.

118. Tsuchiya R, Harada N, Ito T, et al. Malignant tumors in choledochal cysts. Ann Surg. 1977; 186(2): 22-8.
119. Stringer, M. D. Laparoscopic management of choledochal cysts: is a keyhole view missing the big picture? Pediatr Surg Int. 2017 Avr; 33(6): 1-6.
120. Fanny Yeung, Adrian C. H. Fung, Patrick H. Y. Chung, Kenneth K. Y. Wong. Short-term and long-term outcomes after Roux-en-Y hepaticojejunostomy versus hepaticoduodenostomy following laparoscopic excision of choledochal cyst in children. Surg Endosc. 2019 Jul; 34(5): 2172-7.
121. Ohi R, Yaoita S, Kamiyama T, Ibrahim M, Hayashi Y, Chiba T. Surgical treatment of congenital dilatation of the bile duct with special reference to late complications after total excisional operation. J Pediatr Surg. 1990; 25(6): 613-7.
122. Jabłonska. Biliary cysts: etiology, diagnosis and management. World J Gastroenterol. 2012; 18(35): 4801-10.
123. Arkaitz Perfecto Valero, Mikel Gastaca, Prieto M. Biliary cyst of the cystic duct: A case of Todani type VI. Cirugía Española. 2018 Nov; 96 (10): 656 – 666.
124. Giuseppe Vanella, Michiel Bronswijk, Schalk van der Merwe. Needle-knife deroofing of a symptomatic type III choledochal cyst. Endosco. 2019 Dec 52 (6); 1-2.
125. P. A. Lipsett, H. A. Pitt, P. M. Colombani, J. K. Boitnott, and J. L. Cameron. Choledochal cyst disease a changing pattern of presentation. Ann Surg. 1994; 220(5): 644-52.
126. Qian Dong, Buxian Jiang, Hong Zhang, Zhong Jiang, Hongting Lu, Chuanmin Yang, Yu Cheng,and Xiwei Hao. Management Strategy for Congenital Choledochal Cyst withCo-existing Intrahepatic Dilation and Aberrant Bile Duct As Well As Other Complicated Biliary Anomalies. Yonsei Med J. 2006 Dec; 47(6).
127. Hemonta Kr. Dutta. Hepatic lobectomy and mucosectomy of intrahepatic cyst for type IV-A choledochal cyst. J Pediatr Surg. 2012 Jul; 47(2); 2146–2150.
128. J'Y. Mabrut, G. Bozio, C. Hubert, and J.-F. Gigot. Management of congenital bile duct cysts. Dig Surg. 2010; 27(18): 12-8.
129. Sen SS, Menon P, Solanki S, Bhatia A, Sen IM. Acute pancreatitis with Cullen's sign presentation in a case of mixed type I and II choledochal cyst. J Pediatr Surg. 2019 Oct; 54(10): 2187-90.
130. Venkata Vishwanath Reddych, Ashok Kumar, Manas Aggarwal, Kailash Chand Kurdia. Type VI choledochal cyst with gall bladder carcinoma. J Gastrointest Surg. 2019 Dec 29; 12(12): 232715.

131. Marta Garzón-Benavides, Andrea Núñez-Ortiz, Teófilo López-Ruiz, Carmen Cepeda-Franco and LourdesGómez-Izquierdo. Pancreatobiliary maljunction: association with gallbladder cancer. Rev Esp Enferm Dig. 2019 Mar; 111(7); 568-570.
132. Sarath Kumar Narayanana, Yong Chen b, Kannan Laksmi Narasimhan b, Ralph Clinton Cohena. Hepaticoduodenostomy versus hepaticojejunostomy after resection of choledochal cyst: A systematic review and meta-analysis. J Pediatr Surg. 2013 Jul; 48(1); 2336–2342.
133. Vijay Patil, Vijay Kanetkar, Mahesh C. Talpallikar. Hepaticoduodenostomy for Biliary Reconstruction after surgical resection of choledochal Cyst: à 25-Year Experience. Indian J Surg. 2015 Dec; 2(3); 240-244.
134. Yoshinori Hamada, Hiroshi Hamada, Takeshi Shirai, Yusuke Nakamura, Tatsuma Sakaguchi, Hiroaki Yanagimoto, Kentaro Inoue, Masanori Kon. Duodenogastric regurgitation in hepaticoduodenostomy after excision of congenital biliary dilatation (choledochal cyst). J Pediatr Surg. 2017 Oct; 52 (10); 1621-1624.
135. Jesus Morales-Maza, Jorge Humberto Rodríguez-Quintero, Sonia Cortés-Vázquez, Luis Cruz-Benítez. Giant choledochal cyst presenting during third trimester of pregnancy. BMJ Case Rep. 2018 Ju; 13(2); 1-4.
136. Daniel Bennett, Paul McMenamin, Maurizio Pacilli, Tom Clarnette and Ramesh M Nataraja. Novel application of additive manufacturing techniques for paediatric choledochal malformations.J Paeditr Child Health. 2018 Jul; 54 (7): 807-8.
137. Belén Aneiros Castro, ndalecio Cano Novillo, Araceli García Vázquez, Mónica De Miguel Moya. Association between gallbladder agenesis and choledochal cyst: cause or coincidence? BMJ Case Rep. 2019 Jun; 12(6).1-3.
138. Ji Hun Kim, Tae Yong Choi, Jae Ho Han, Byung Moo Yoo, Jin Hong Kim, Jeong Hong, Myung Wook Kim, Wook Hwan Kim. Risk Factors of Postoperative Anastomotic Stricture after excision of Choledochal Cysts with Hepaticojejunostomy. J Gastrointest Surg. 2008 May; 12(5): 822-8.
139. Takanori Aota, Shoji Kubo, Shigekazu Takemura, Shogo Tanaka, Ryosuke Amano, Kenjiro Kimura, Sadaaki Yamazoe, Hiroji Shinkawa, Go Ohira, Toshihiko Shibata, Masaki Horiike. Long-term outcomes after biliary diversion operation for pancreaticobiliary maljunction in adult patients.Ann Gastroenterol Surg. 2019 Jan; 3 (1); 217–223.

140. Soo Young Oh, Jae Hyun Kwon, and Shin Hwang. Development of adenocarcinoma at the remnant intrapancreatic cyst 16 years after resection of the choledochal cyst. Ann Hepatobiliary Pancreat Surg. 2019; 23 (2): 192-196.
141. Lili Wang, Xiaomei Ma1, Dongdong Chen, Jialiang Ren, Hua Cheng, Gang Huang, Rong Wang and Jiarong Cheng. Primary congenital choledochal cyst with squamous cell carcinoma: a case report. J Int Med Res. 2020 Sep 48(9) 1–6.
142. Ahlem Lahmar, Sadri Ben Abid, Mohamed Nafaa Arfa, Rached Bayar, Mohamed Tahar Khalfallah, Sabah Mzabi Regaya. Metachronous cancer of gallbladder and pancreas with pancreatobiliary maljunction. World J Gastrointest Surg. 2010 Ap; 2 (4): 143-146.

Part 2: Pancreatic ducts anomalies

1. Gutta A1, Fogel E1, Sherman S1. Identification and management of pancreas divisum Expert Rev Gastroenterol Hepatol. 2019 Nov; 13(11): 1089-1105.
2. Kozu T, Suda K, Toki F. Pancreatic development and anatomical variation. Gastrointestinal endoscopy clinics of North America. 1995 Jan; 5(1): 1-30.
3. Smanio T. Proposed nomenclature and classification of the human pancreatic ducts and duodenal papillae. Study based on 200 post mortems. International surgery. 1969 Aug; 52(2): 125-41.
4. Stimec B, Bulajic M, Korneti V, et al. Ductal morphometry of ventral pancreas in pancreas divisum. Comparison between clinical and anatomical results. The Italian journal of gastroenterology. 1996 Feb-Mar; 28(2): 76-80. PubMed PMID: 8781998.
5. Bernard JP, Sahel J, Giovannini M, et al. Pancreas divisum is a probable cause of acute pancreatitis: a report of 137 cases. Pancreas. 1990 May; 5(3): 248-54. PubMed PMID: 2343039.
6. Liao Z, Gao R, Wang W, et al. A systematic review on endoscopic detection rate, endotherapy, and surgery for pancreas divisum. Endoscopy. 2009 May; 41(5): 439-44. doi: 10.1055/s-0029-1214505. PubMed PMID: 19337962.
7. Bulow R, Simon P, Thiel R, et al. Anatomic variants of the pancreatic duct and their clinical relevance: an MR-guided study in the general population. European radiology. 2014 Dec; 24(12): 3142-9. doi: 10.1007/s00330-014-3359-7. PubMed PMID: 25120204.

8. Suga T, Nakagawa T, Miyakawa H, et al. Clinical Features of Patients with Pancreas Divisum. 1994; 6(1): 80-86. doi: 10.1111/j.1443-1661.1994.tb00668.x.
9. Varshney S., Johnson C.D. Surgery for pancreas divisum Ann. R. Coll. Surg. Engl. 2002; 84 (3): 166-169.
10. Kamisawa T, Koike M, Okamoto A. Embryology of the pancreatic duct system. Digestion. 1999 Mar-Apr; 60(2): 161-5. doi: 10.1159/000007642. PubMed PMID: 10095158.
11. Kamisawa T, Takuma K, Egawa N, et al. A new embryological theory of the pancreatic duct system. Digestive surgery. 2010; 27(2): 132-6. doi: 10.1159/000286906. PubMed PMID: 20551658.
12. MacCarty RL, Stephens DH, Brown AL, Jr., et al. Retrograde pancreatography in autopsy specimens. The American journal of roentgenology, radium therapy, and nuclear medicine. 1975 Feb; 123(2): 359-66. PubMed PMID: 1115312.
13. Kamisawa T, Egawa N, Tu Y, et al. Pancreatographic investigation of embryology of complete and incomplete pancreas divisum. Pancreas. 2007 Jan; 34(1): 96-102. doi: 10.1097/01.mpa.0000240607.49183.7e. PubMed PMID: 17198190.
14. Moreira VF, Merono E, Ledo L, et al. Incomplete pancreas divisum. Gastrointestinal endoscopy. 1991 Jan-Feb; 37(1): 104-5. PubMed PMID: 2004672.
15. Tulassay Z, Papp J, Farkas IE. Diagnostic aspects of incomplete pancreas divisum. Gastrointestinal endoscopy. 1986 Dec; 32(6): 428. PubMed PMID: 3803848.
16. Zyromski NJ, Sandoval JA, Pitt HA, et al. Annular pancreas: dramatic differences between children and adults. Journal of the American College of Surgeons. 2008 May; 206(5): 1019-25; discussion 1025-7. doi: 10.1016/j.jamcollsurg.2007.12.009. PubMed PMID: 18471747.
17. Lehman GA, O'Connor KW. Coexistence of annular pancreas and pancreas divisum-ERCP diagnosis. Gastrointestinal endoscopy. 1985 Feb; 31(1): 25-8. PubMed PMID: 3979764.
18. Sandrasegaran K, Patel A, Fogel EL, et al. Annular pancreas in adults. AJR American journal of roentgenology. 2009 Aug; 193(2): 455-60. doi: 10.2214/ajr.08.1596. PubMed PMID: 19620443.
19. Gromski MA, Lehman GA, Zyromski NJ, et al. Annular pancreas: endoscopic and pancreatographic findings from a tertiary referral ERCP center. Gastrointestinal endoscopy. 2018 Sep 18. doi: 10.1016/j.gie.2018.09.008. PubMed PMID: 30240880; eng.
20. Cao J, Wang L, Zou X. Coexistence of Complete Pancreas Divisum and Anomalous Pancreaticobiliary Junction in a Patient With Type IA

Choledochal Cyst. Clinical gastroenterology and hepatology: the official clinical practice journal of the American Gastroenterological Association. 2018 Aug 2. doi: 10.1016/j.cgh.2018.07.036. PubMed PMID: 30077786; eng.

21. Ng JW, Wong MK, Huang J, et al. Incomplete pancreas divisum associated with abnormal junction of pancreaticobiliary duct system. Gastrointestinal endoscopy. 1992 Jan-Feb; 38(1): 105-6. PubMed PMID: 1612369; eng.
22. Patidar Y, Agarwal N, Gupta S, et al. Choledochocele with pancreas divisum: A rare cooccurrence diagnosed on magnetic resonance cholangiopancreatography. World journal of radiology. 2013 Jul 28; 5(7): 264-6. doi: 10.4329/wjr.v5.i7.264. PubMed PMID: 23908697; eng.
23. Ransom-Rodriguez A, Blachman-Braun R, Sanchez-Garcia Ramos E, et al. A rare case of choledochal cyst with pancreas divisum: case presentation and literature review. Annals of hepato-biliary-pancreatic surgery. 2017 Feb; 21(1): 52-56. doi: 10.14701/ahbps.2017.21.1.52. PubMed PMID: 28317046; PubMed Central PMCID: PMCPMC5353911; eng.
24. Sanada Y, Sakuma Y, Sata N. Embryological etiology of pancreaticobiliary system predicted from pancreaticobiliary maljunction with incomplete pancreatic divisum: a case report. BMC surgery. 2018 Aug 2; 18(1): 50. doi: 10.1186/s12893-018-0385-4. PubMed PMID: 30068344; PubMed Central PMCID: PMCPMC6090945; eng.
25. Adibelli ZH, Adatepe M, Isayeva L, et al. Pancreas divisum: A risk factor for pancreaticobiliary tumors - an analysis of 1628 MR cholangiography examinations. Diagnostic and interventional imaging. 2017 Feb; 98(2): 141-147. doi: 10.1016/j.diii.2016.08.004. PubMed PMID: 27616039; eng.
26. Lehman GA, Kopecky KK, Rogge JD. Partial pancreatic agenesis combined with pancreas divisum and duodenum reflexum. Gastrointestinal endoscopy. 1987 Dec; 33(6): 445-8. PubMed PMID: 3443265; eng.
27. Canto MI, Harinck F, Hruban RH, et al. International Cancer of the Pancreas Screening (CAPS) Consortium summit on the management of patients with increased risk for familial pancreatic cancer. Gut. 2013; 62(3): 339-347. doi: 10.1136/gutjnl-2012-303108.
28. Nishi T, Kawabata Y, Ishikawa N, et al. Intraductal papillary mucinous carcinoma of the pancreas associated with pancreas divisum: a case report and review of the literature. BMC

gastroenterology. 2015 Jul 8; 15: 78. doi: 10.1186/s12876-015-0313-3. PubMed PMID: 26152300; PubMed Central PMCID: PMCPMC4495851; eng.
29. Madura JA. Pancreas divisum: stenosis of the dorsally dominant pancreatic duct. A surgically correctable lesion. American journal of surgery. 1986 Jun; 151(6): 742-5. PubMed PMID: 3717505; eng.
30. Warshaw AL, Simeone JF, Schapiro RH, et al. Evaluation and treatment of the dominant dorsal duct syndrome (pancreas divisum redefined). American journal of surgery. 1990 Jan; 159(1): 59-64; discussion 64-66. PubMed PMID: 2403764; eng.
31. Staritz M, Meyer zum Buschenfelde KH. Elevated pressure in the dorsal part of pancreas divisum: the cause of chronic pancreatitis? Pancreas. 1988; 3(1): 108-10. PubMed PMID: 3362837; eng.
32. Cotton PB. Pancreas divisum--curiosity or culprit? Gastroenterology. 1985 Dec; 89(6): 1431-5. PubMed PMID: 4054536; eng.
33. Cotton PB. Congenital anomaly of pancreas divisum as cause of obstructive pain and pancreatitis. 1980; 21(2): 105-114. doi: 10.1136/gut.21.2.105 %J Gut.
34. Guirat A, Abid M, Ben Amar M, Rebai W, Beyrouti MI. Pancréas divisum [Pancreas divisum]. Presse Med. 2009; 38(9): 1353-1359. doi: 10.1016/j.lpm.2008.05.024
35. Bertin C, Pelletier AL, Vullierme MP, et al. Pancreas divisum is not a cause of pancreatitis by itself but acts as a partner of genetic mutations. The American journal of gastroenterology. 2012 Feb; 107(2): 311-7. doi: 10.1038/ajg.2011.424. PubMed PMID: 22158025; eng.
36. Delhaye M, Engelholm L, Cremer M. Pancreas divisum: congenital anatomic variant or anomaly? Contribution of endoscopic retrograde dorsal pancreatography. Gastroenterology. 1985 Nov; 89(5): 951-8. PubMed PMID: 4043675; eng.
37. Barthet M, Valantin V, Spinosa S, et al. Clinical course and morphological features of chronic calcifying pancreatitis associated with pancreas divisum. European Journal of Gastroenterology & Hepatology. 1995; 7(10): 993-998. PubMed PMID: 00042737-199510000-00016.
38. Spicak J, Poulova P, Plucnarova J, et al. Pancreas divisum does not modify the natural course of chronic pancreatitis [journal article]. Journal of Gastroenterology. 2007 February 01; 42(2): 135-139. doi: 10.1007/s00535-006-1976-x.
39. Dhar A, Goenka MK, Kochhar R, et al. Pancrease divisum: five years' experience in a teaching hospital. Indian journal of gastroenterology:

official journal of the Indian Society of Gastroenterology. 1996 Jan; 15(1): 7-9. PubMed PMID: 8840617; eng.
40. Morgan DE, Logan K, Baron TH, et al. Pancreas divisum: implications for diagnostic and therapeutic pancreatography. AJR American journal of roentgenology. 1999 Jul; 173(1): 193-8. doi: 10.2214/ajr.173.1.10397125. PubMed PMID: 10397125; eng.
41. Wang DB, Yu J, Fulcher AS, et al. Pancreatitis in patients with pancreas divisum: imaging features at MRI and MRCP. World journal of gastroenterology. 2013 Aug 14; 19(30): 4907-16. doi: 10.3748/wjg.v19.i30.4907. PubMed PMID: 23946595; PubMed Central PMCID: PMCPMC3740420; eng.
42. Lin TK, Abu-El-Haija M, Nathan JD, et al. Pancreas Divisum in Pediatric Acute Recurrent and Chronic Pancreatitis: Report From INSPPIRE. Journal of clinical gastroenterology. 2018 Jun 2. doi: 10.1097/mcg.0000000000001063. PubMed PMID: 29864067; eng.
43. Benage D, McHenry R, Hawes RH, et al. Minor papilla cannulation and dorsal ductography in pancreas divisum. Gastrointestinal endoscopy. 1990 Nov-Dec; 36(6): 553-7. PubMed PMID: 2279641; eng.
44. Borak GD, Romagnuolo J, Alsolaiman M, et al. Long-term clinical outcomes after endoscopic minor papilla therapy in symptomatic patients with pancreas divisum. Pancreas. 2009 Nov; 38(8): 903-6. doi: 10.1097/MPA.0b013e3181b2bc03. PubMed PMID: 19672208; eng.
45. Chacko LN, Chen YK, Shah RJ. Clinical outcomes and nonendoscopic interventions after minor papilla endotherapy in patients with symptomatic pancreas divisum. Gastrointestinal endoscopy. 2008 Oct; 68(4): 667-73. doi: 10.1016/j.gie.2008.01.025. PubMed PMID: 18436218; eng.
46. Lans JI, Geenen JE, Johanson JF, et al. Endoscopic therapy in patients with pancreas divisum and acute pancreatitis: a prospective, randomized, controlled clinical trial. Gastrointestinal endoscopy. 1992 Jul-Aug; 38(4): 430-4. PubMed PMID: 1511816; eng.
47. Lehman GA, Sherman S, Nisi R, et al. Pancreas divisum: results of minor papilla sphincterotomy. Gastrointestinal endoscopy. 1993 Jan-Feb; 39(1): 1-8. PubMed PMID: 8454127; eng.
48. Heyries L, Barthet M, Delvasto C, et al. Long-term results of endoscopic management of pancreas divisum with recurrent acute pancreatitis. Gastrointestinal endoscopy. 2002 Mar; 55(3): 376-81. doi: 10.1067/mge.2002.121602. PubMed PMID: 11868012; eng.

49. Keith RG, Shapero TF, Saibil FG, et al. Dorsal duct sphincterotomy is effective long-term treatment of acute pancreatitis associated with pancreas divisum. Surgery. 1989 Oct; 106(4): 660-6; discussion 666-7. PubMed PMID: 2799640; eng.
50. Kwan V, Loh SM, Walsh PR, et al. Minor papilla sphincterotomy for pancreatitis due to pancreas divisum. ANZ journal of surgery. 2008 Apr; 78(4): 257-61. doi: 10.1111/j.1445-2197.2008.04431.x. PubMed PMID: 18366396; eng.
51. Siegel JH, Ben-Zvi JS, Pullano W, et al. Effectiveness of endoscopic drainage for pancreas divisum: endoscopic and surgical results in 31 patients. Endoscopy. 1990 May; 22(3): 129-33. doi: 10.1055/s-2007-1010727. PubMed PMID: 2103724; eng.
52. Klein SD, Affronti JP. Pancreas divisum, an evidence-based review: part I, pathophysiology. Gastrointestinal endoscopy. 2004 Sep; 60(3): 419-25. PubMed PMID: 15332034; eng.
53. Garg PK, Khajuria R, Kabra M, et al. Association of SPINK1 gene mutation and CFTR gene polymorphisms in patients with pancreas divisum presenting with idiopathic pancreatitis. Journal of clinical gastroenterology. 2009 Oct; 43(9): 848-52. doi: 10.1097/MCG.0b013e3181a4e772. PubMed PMID: 19593166; eng.
54. Gelrud A, Sheth S, Banerjee S, et al. Analysis of cystic fibrosis gener product (CFTR) function in patients with pancreas divisum and recurrent acute pancreatitis. The American journal of gastroenterology. 2004 Aug; 99(8): 1557-62. doi: 10.1111/j.1572-0241.2004.30834.x. PubMed PMID: 15307877; eng.
55. Choudari CP, Imperiale TF, Sherman S, et al. Risk of Pancreatitis with Mutation of the Cystic Fibrosis Gene [Original Contribution]. American Journal Of Gastroenterology. 2004 07/01/online; 99: 1358. doi: 10.1111/j.1572-0241.2004.30655.x.
56. Bhatia E, Choudhuri G, Sikora SS, et al. Tropical calcific pancreatitis: strong association with SPINK1 trypsin inhibitor mutations. Gastroenterology. 2002 Oct; 123(4): 1020-5. PubMed PMID: 12360463; eng.
57. Cohn JA, Friedman KJ, Noone PG, et al. Relation between mutations of the cystic fibrosis gene and idiopathic pancreatitis. The New England journal of medicine. 1998 Sep 3; 339(10): 653-8. doi: 10.1056/nejm199809033391002. PubMed PMID: 9725922; eng.
58. Witt H, Luck W, Hennies HC, et al. Mutations in the gene encoding the serine protease inhibitor, Kazal type 1 are associated with chronic

pancreatitis. Nature genetics. 2000 Jun; 25(2): 213-6. doi: 10.1038/76088. PubMed PMID: 10835640; eng.

59. Lin TK, Abu-El-Haija M, Nathan JD, et al. Pancreas Divisum in Pediatric Acute Recurrent and Chronic Pancreatitis: Report From INSPPIRE. Journal of clinical gastroenterology. 2019 Jul; 53(6): e232-e238. doi: 10.1097/mcg.0000000000001063. PubMed PMID: 29864067; PubMed Central PMCID: PMCPMC6275137; eng.

60. Adike A, El Kurdi BI, Gaddam S, et al. Pancreatitis in Patients With Pancreas Divisum. Pancreas. 2017; 46(10): e80-e81. doi: 10.1097/mpa.0000000000000938. PubMed PMID: 00006676-201711000-00026.

61. Liguory C., Lefebvre J.F., Canard J.M., Bonnel D., Fritsch J., Etienne J.P. Pancreas divisum: clinical and therapeutic study in man. Apropos of 87 cases Gastroenterol. Clin. Biol. 1986; 10 (12): 820-825.

62. Coyle W.J., Pineau B.C., Tarnasky P.R., Knapple W.L., Aabakken L., Hoffman B.J., and al. Evaluation of unexplained acute and acute recurrent pancreatitis using endoscopic retrograde cholangiopancreatography, sphincter of Oddi manometry and endoscopic ultrasound Endoscopy 2002; 34 (8): 617-623.

63. Takuma K, Kamisawa T, Hara S, et al. Etiology of recurrent acute pancreatitis, with special emphasis on pancreaticobiliary malformation. Advances in medical sciences. 2012; 57(2): 244-50. doi: 10.2478/v10039-012-0041-7. PubMed PMID: 23183766; eng.

64. Kim M.H., Lee S.S., Kim C.D., Lee S.K., Kim H.J., Park H.J. Incomplete pancreas divisum: is it merely a normal anatomic variant without clinical implications? Endoscopy 2001; 33 (9): 778-785.

65. Barthet M., Valantin V., Spinosa S., Bernard J.P., Sahel J. Clinical course and morphological features of chronic calcifying pancreatitis associated with pancreas divisum Eur. J. Gastroenterol. Hepatol. 1995; 7 (10): 993-998.

66. Browder W., Gravois E., Vega P., Ertan A. Obstructing pseudocyst of the duct of Santorini in pancreas divisum Am. J. Gastroenterol. 1987; 82 (3): 258-261.

67. Simmons T.C., Henderson D.R., Gletten F. Pancreatic abscess associated with pancreas divisum J. Natl. Med. Assoc. 1988; 80 (4): 453-455457-458.

68. Vazquez-Iglesias J.L., Durana J.A., Yanez J., Rodriguez H., Garcia-Vallejo L., Arnal F. Santorinirrhage: hemosuccus pancreaticus in pancreas divisum Am. J. Gastroenterol. 1988; 83 (8): 876-878.

69. Asayama Y, Fang W, Stolpen A, et al. Detectability of pancreas divisum in patients with acute pancreatitis on multi-detector row computed tomography. Emergency radiology. 2012 Apr; 19(2): 121-5. doi: 10.1007/s10140-011-1008-x. PubMed PMID: 22167339; eng.
70. Kushnir VM, Wani SB, Fowler K, et al. Sensitivity of endoscopic ultrasound, multidetector computed tomography, and magnetic resonance cholangiopancreatography in the diagnosis of pancreas divisum: a tertiary center experience. Pancreas. 2013 Apr; 42(3): 436-41.
doi: 10.1097/MPA.0b013e31826c711a. PubMed PMID: 23211370; PubMed Central PMCID: PMCPMC3928633; eng.
71. Lindstrom E, Ihse I. Dynamic CT scanning of pancreatic duct after secretin provocation in pancreas divisum. Digestive diseases and sciences. 1990 Nov; 35(11): 1371-6. PubMed PMID: 1699712; eng.
72. Rustagi T, Njei B. Magnetic resonance cholangiopancreatography in the diagnosis of pancreas divisum: a systematic review and meta-analysis. Pancreas. 2014 Aug; 43(6): 823-8. doi: 10.1097/mpa.0000000000000143. PubMed PMID: 24743381; eng.
73. Shen Z, Munker S, Zhou B, et al. The Accuracies of Diagnosing Pancreas Divisum by Magnetic Resonance Cholangiopancreatography and Endoscopic Ultrasound: A Systematic Review and Meta-analysis. Scientific reports. 2016 Oct 13; 6: 35389. doi: 10.1038/srep35389. PubMed PMID: 27734952; PubMed Central PMCID: PMCPMC5062127; eng.
74. Wan J, Ouyang Y, Yu C, et al. Comparison of EUS with MRCP in idiopathic acute pancreatitis: a systematic review and meta-analysis. Gastrointestinal endoscopy. 2018 May; 87(5): 1180-1188.e9. doi: 10.1016/j.gie.2017.11.028. PubMed PMID: 29225082; eng.
75. Boninsegna E, Manfredi R, Ventriglia A, et al. Santorinicele: secretin-enhanced magnetic resonance cholangiopancreatography findings before and after minor papilla sphincterotomy. European radiology. 2015 Aug; 25(8): 2437-44. doi: 10.1007/s00330-015-3644-0. PubMed PMID: 25693665; eng.
76. Manfredi R, Brizi MG, Costamagna G, et al. Pancreas divisum and santorinicele: assessment by dynamic magnetic resonance cholangiopancreatography during secretin stimulation. La Radiologia medica. 2002 Jan-Feb; 103(1-2): 55-64.
77. Bhutani MS, Hoffmann BJ. Diagnostic of pancreas divisum by endoscopic ultrasonography. Endoscopy 1999; 39: 312.
78. Lai R, Freeman ML, Cass OW, et al. Accurate diagnosis of pancreas divisum by lineararray endoscopic ultrasonography. Endoscopy. 2004

Aug; 36(8): 705-9. doi: 10.1055/s-2004-825663. PubMed PMID: 15280976; eng.
79. Rana SS, Bhasin DK, Sharma V, et al. Role of endoscopic ultrasound in the diagnosis of pancreas divisum. Endoscopic ultrasound. 2013 Jan-Mar; 2(1): 7-10. doi: 10.7178/eus.04.003. PubMed PMID: 24949360; PubMed Central PMCID: PMCPMC4062234; eng.
80. Catalano MF RM, Geenen JE, et al. Pancreatic endotherapy of pancreas divisum (PDIV): Response based on clinical presentation and results of secretin stimulated endoscopic ultrasound: (S-EUS). Gastrointestinal endoscopy. 2001; 53(5): AB133. doi: 10.1016/S0016-5107(01)80267-4.
81. Sharma M, Pathak A, Rameshbabu CS, et al. Imaging of pancreas divisum by linear-array endoscopic ultrasonography. Endoscopic ultrasound. 2016 Jan-Feb; 5(1): 21-9. doi: 10.4103/2303-9027.175878. PubMed PMID: 26879163; PubMed Central PMCID: PMCPMC4770618; eng.
82. Lehman GA, Sherman S. Pancreas divisum. Diagnosis, clinical significance, and management alternatives. Gastrointestinal endoscopy clinics of North America. 1995 Jan; 5(1): 145-70. PubMed PMID: 7728342; eng.
83. Lehman GA, Sherman S. Diagnosis and therapy of pancreas divisum. Gastrointestinal endoscopy clinics of North America. 1998 Jan; 8(1): 55-77. PubMed PMID: 9405751; eng.
84. McCarthy J, Fumo D, Geenen JE. Pancreas divisum: a new method for cannulating the accessory papilla. Gastrointestinal endoscopy. 1987 Dec; 33(6): 440-2. PubMed PMID: 3443264; eng.
85. O'Connor KW, Lehman GA. An improved technique for accessory papilla cannulation in pancreas divisum. Gastrointestinal endoscopy. 1985 Feb; 31(1): 13-7. PubMed PMID: 3979760; eng.
86. Ertan A. Long-term results after endoscopic pancreatic stent placement without pancreatic papillotomy in acute recurrent pancreatitis due to pancreas divisum. Gastrointestinal endoscopy. 2000 Jul; 52(1): 9-14. doi: 10.1067/mge.2000.106311. PubMed PMID: 10882955; eng.
87. Jacob L, Geenen JE, Catalano MF, et al. Clinical presentation and short-term outcome of endoscopic therapy of patients with symptomatic incomplete pancreas divisum. Gastrointestinal endoscopy. 1999 Jan; 49(1): 53-7. PubMed PMID: 9869723; eng.
88. Devereaux BM, Fein S, Purich E, et al. A new synthetic porcine secretin for facilitation of cannulation of the dorsal pancreatic duct at ERCP in patients with pancreas divisum: a multicenter, randomized,

double-blind comparative study. Gastrointestinal endoscopy. 2003 May; 57(6): 643-7.
doi: 10.1067/mge.2003.195. PubMed PMID: 12709690; eng.
89. Park SH, de Bellis M, McHenry L, et al. Use of methylene blue to identify the minor papilla or its orifice in patients with pancreas divisum. Gastrointestinal endoscopy. 2003 Mar; 57(3): 358-63. doi: 10.1067/mge.2003.110. PubMed PMID: 12612516; eng.
90. Gerke H, Byrne MF, Stiffler HL, et al. Outcome of endoscopic minor papillotomy in patients with symptomatic pancreas divisum. JOP: Journal of the pancreas. 2004 May; 5(3): 122-31. PubMed PMID: 15138333; eng.
91. Moffatt DC, Cote GA, Avula H, et al. Risk factors for ERCP-related complications in patients with pancreas divisum: a retrospective study. Gastrointestinal endoscopy. 2011 May; 73(5): 963-70. doi: 10.1016/j.gie.2010.12.035. PubMed PMID: 21392753; eng.
92. Freeman ML, DiSario JA, Nelson DB, et al. Risk factors for post-ERCP pancreatitis: a prospective, multicenter study. Gastrointestinal endoscopy. 2001 Oct; 54(4): 425-34. PubMed PMID: 11577302; eng.
93. Sofuni A, Maguchi H, Itoi T, et al. Prophylaxis of post-endoscopic retrograde cholangiopancreatography pancreatitis by an endoscopic pancreatic spontaneous dislodgement stent. Clinical gastroenterology and hepatology: the official clinical practice journal of the American Gastroenterological Association. 2007 Nov; 5(11): 1339-46. doi: 10.1016/j.cgh.2007.07.008. PubMed PMID: 17981247; eng.
94. Sherman S, Eversman D, Fogel E, et al. Sphincter of oddi dysfunction (SOD): Needleknife pancreatobiliary sphincterotomy over pancreatic stent (NKOPS) has a lower postprocedure pancreatitis rate than pull-type biliary sphincterotomy (BES). Gastrointestinal endoscopy. 1997; 45(4): AB148. doi: 10.1016/S0016-5107(97)80496-8.
95. Tarnasky PR. Mechanical prevention of post-ERCP pancreatitis by pancreatic stents: results, techniques, and indications. JOP: Journal of the Pancreas. 2003 Jan; 4(1): 58-67. PubMed PMID: 12555017; eng.
96. Rashdan A, Fogel EL, McHenry L, Jr., et al. Improved stent characteristics for prophylaxis of post-ERCP pancreatitis. Clinical gastroenterology and hepatology: the official clinical practice journal of the American Gastroenterological Association. 2004 Apr; 2(4): 322-9. PubMed PMID: 15067627; eng.
97. Bhandari S, Sharma A, Bathini R, Maydeo A. Endoscopic management of internally migrated pancreatic duct stents (with video). Indian J Gastroenterol. 2016; 35(2): 91-100. doi: 10.1007/s12664-016-0638-z.

98. Kerdsirichairat T, Attam R, Arain M, et al. Urgent ERCP with pancreatic stent placement or replacement for salvage of post-ERCP pancreatitis. Endoscopy. 2014 Dec; 46(12): 1085-94. doi: 10.1055/s-0034-1377750. PubMed PMID: 25216326; eng.
99. Elmunzer BJ, Scheiman JM, Lehman GA, et al. A randomized trial of rectal indomethacin to prevent post-ERCP pancreatitis. The New England journal of medicine. 2012 Apr 12; 366(15): 1414-22. doi: 10.1056/NEJMoa1111103. PubMed PMID: 22494121; PubMed Central PMCID: PMCPMC3339271; eng.
100. Garg R, Mohan BP, Krishnamoorthi R, et al. Pre-endoscopic retrograde cholangiopancreatography (ERCP) administration of rectal indomethacin in unselected patients to reduce post-ERCP pancreatitis: A systematic review and meta-analysis. Indian journal of gastroenterology: official journal of the Indian Society of Gastroenterology. 2018 Mar; 37(2): 120-126. doi: 10.1007/s12664-018-0841-1. PubMed PMID: 29619673; eng.
101. Inamdar S, Han D, Passi M, et al. Rectal indomethacin is protective against post-ERCP pancreatitis in high-risk patients but not average-risk patients: a systematic review and meta-analysis. Gastrointestinal endoscopy. 2017 Jan; 85(1): 67-75. doi: 10.1016/j.gie.2016.08.034. PubMed PMID: 27612923; eng.
102. Lyu Y, Cheng Y, Wang B, et al. What is impact of nonsteroidal anti-inflammatory drugs in the prevention of post-endoscopic retrograde cholangiopancreatography pancreatitis: a meta-analysis of randomized controlled trials. BMC gastroenterology. 2018 Jul 4; 18(1): 106. doi: 10.1186/s12876-018-0837-4. PubMed PMID: 29973142; PubMed Central PMCID: PMCPMC6032784; eng.
103. Buxbaum J, Yan A, Yeh K, et al. Aggressive hydration with lactated Ringer's solution reduces pancreatitis after endoscopic retrograde cholangiopancreatography. Clinical gastroenterology and hepatology: the official clinical practice journal of the American Gastroenterological Association. 2014 Feb; 12(2): 303-7.e1. doi: 10.1016/j.cgh.2013.07.026. PubMed PMID: 23920031; PubMed Central PMCID: PMCPMC3879172; eng.
104. Yamamoto N, Isayama H, Sasahira N, et al. Endoscopic minor papilla balloon dilation for the treatment of symptomatic pancreas divisum. Pancreas. 2014 Aug; 43(6): 927-30. doi: 10.1097/mpa.0000000000000148. PubMed PMID: 24826883; eng.
105. Guelrud M, Mendoza S, Viera L, Gelrud D. Somatostatin prevents acute pancreatitis after pancreatic duct sphincter hydrostatic balloon

dilation in patients with idiopathic recurrent pancreatitis. Gastrointest Endosc 1991; 37: 44-7.
106. Lu Y, Xu B, Chen L, Bie LK, Gong B. Endoscopic intervention through endoscopic retrograde cholangiopancreatography in the management of symptomatic pancreas divisum: a long-term follow-up study. Gut Liver 2016; 10: 476–482.
107. Johanson JF, Schmalz MJ, Geenen JE. Incidence and risk factors for biliary and pancreatic stent migration. Gastrointestinal endoscopy. 1992 May-Jun; 38(3): 341-6. PubMed PMID: 1607087; eng.
108. Ikenberry SO, Sherman S, Hawes RH, et al. The occlusion rate of pancreatic stents. Gastrointestinal endoscopy. 1994 Sep-Oct; 40(5): 611-3. PubMed PMID: 7988829; eng.
109. Smith MT, Sherman S, Ikenberry SO, et al. Alterations in pancreatic ductal morphology following polyethylene pancreatic stent therapy. Gastrointestinal endoscopy. 1996 Sep; 44(3): 268-75. PubMed PMID: 8885345; eng.
110. Kozarek RA. Pancreatic stents can induce ductal changes consistent with chronic pancreatitis. Gastrointestinal endoscopy. 1990 Mar-Apr; 36(2): 93-5. PubMed PMID: 2335298; eng.
111. Sherman S, Hawes RH, Savides TJ, et al. Stent-induced pancreatic ductal and parenchymal changes: correlation of endoscopic ultrasound with ERCP. Gastrointestinal endoscopy. 1996 Sep; 44(3): 276-82. PubMed PMID: 8885346; eng.
112. Ferri V, Vicente E and Quijano Y et al., Diagnosis and treatment of pancreas divisum: A literature review, Hepatobiliary & Pancreatic Diseases International. 2019 Aug; 18(4): 332-336. doi: 10.1016/j.hbpd.2019.05.004. PubMed PMID: 31155429, eng.
113. Mariani A, Di Leo M, Petrone MC, et al. Outcome of endotherapy for pancreas divisum in patients with acute recurrent pancreatitis. World journal of gastroenterology. 2014 Dec 14; 20(46): 17468-75. doi: 10.3748/wjg.v20.i46.17468. PubMed PMID: 25516660; PubMed Central PMCID: PMCPMC4265607; eng.
114. Kanth R, Samji NS, Inaganti A, et al. Endotherapy in symptomatic pancreas divisum: a systematic review. Pancreatology: official journal of the International Association of Pancreatology (IAP) [et al.]. 2014 Jul-Aug; 14(4): 244-50. doi: 10.1016/j.pan.2014.05.796. PubMed PMID: 25062871; eng.
115. Michailidis L, Aslam B, Grigorian A, et al. The efficacy of endoscopic therapy for pancreas divisum: a meta-analysis. Annals of gastroenterology. 2017; 30(5): 550-558.

doi: 10.20524/aog.2017.0159. PubMed PMID: 28845111; PubMed Central PMCID: PMCPMC5566776; eng.
116. Hafezi M, Mayschak B, Probst P, et al. A systematic review and quantitative analysis of different therapies for pancreas divisum. American journal of surgery. 2017 Sep; 214(3): 525-537. doi: 10.1016/j.amjsurg.2016.12.025. PubMed PMID: 28110914; eng.
117. Tierney J, Bhutiani N, Brown AN, Richey JS, Bahr MH, Vitale GC. Identifying Factors Predicting Response to Endoscopic Management of Chronic Pancreatitis Secondary to Pancreas Divisum. J Gastrointest Surg. 2020; 24(3): 585-589. doi: 10.1007/s11605-019-04122-2.
118. Boerma D, Huibregtse K, Gulik TM, Rauws EA, Obertop H, Gouma DJ. Long-term outcome of endoscopic stent placement for chronic pancreatitis associated with pancreas divisum. Endoscopy. 2000; 32(6): 452–6.
119. Bradley EL, 3rd, Stephan RN. Accessory duct sphincteroplasty is preferred for long-term prevention of recurrent acute pancreatitis in patients with pancreas divisum. Journal of the American College of Surgeons. 1996 Jul; 183(1): 65-70. PubMed PMID: 8673310; eng.
120. Anderson MA, Akshintala V, Albers KM, et al. Mechanism, assessment and management of pain in chronic pancreatitis: Recommendations of a multidisciplinary study group. Pancreatology: official journal of the International Association of Pancreatology (IAP) [et al.]. 2016 Jan-Feb; 16(1): 83-94.
doi: 10.1016/j.pan.2015.10.015. PubMed PMID: 26620965; PubMed Central PMCID: PMCPMC4761301; eng.
121. Pappas SG, Pilgrim CH, Keim R, et al. The Frey procedure for chronic pancreatitis secondary to pancreas divisum. JAMA surgery. 2013 Nov; 148(11): 1057-62. doi: 10.1001/jamasurg.2013.3728. PubMed PMID: 24005579; eng.
122. Skorzewska M, Romanowicz T, Mielko J, et al. Frey operation for chronic pancreatitis associated with pancreas divisum: case report and review of the literature. Przeglad gastroenterologiczny. 2014; 9(3): 175-8. doi: 10.5114/pg.2014.43581. PubMed PMID: 25097717; PubMed Central PMCID: PMCPMC4110366; eng.
123. Cameron JL, Sandone C: Atlas de chirurgie gastro-intestinale, éd 2, vol 2, Shelton, Cann, 2012, PMPH-Etats-Unis.
124. Schneider L, Müller E, Hinz U, Grenacher L, Büchler MW, Werner J. Pancreas divisum: a differentiated surgical approach in symptomatic patients. World J Surg 2011; 35: 1360–1366.

125. Schnelldorfer T, Adams DB. Outcome after lateral pancreaticojejunostomy in patients with chronic pancreatitis associated with pancreas divisum. Am Surg 2003; 69: 1041–1046.
126. Vicente E, Quijano Y, Ferri V, Ielpo B, Diaz E, Caruso R et al. Pancreas divisum: duodenal-preserving resection of the head of the pancreas and pancreatic head. Resection wit second-portion duodenectomy. Cir Esp 2014; 92: 1032.
127. Andersen DK, Frey CF. The evolution of the surgical treatment of chronic pancreatitis. Ann Surg 2010; 251: 18–32.
128. Beger HG, Siech M, Poch B. Duodenum-preserving total pancreatic head resection: an organ-sparing operation technique for cystic neoplasms and non-invasive malignant tumors. Chirurg 2013; 84: 412–420.
129. Frey CF, Smith GJ. Description and rationale of a new operation for chronic pancreatitis. Pancreas 1987; 2: 701–707
130. Gloor B, Friess H, Uhl W, Büchler MW. A modified technique of the Beger and Frey procedure in patients with chronic pancreatitis. Dig Surg 2001; 18: 21–25.
131. Nakao A. Pancreatic head resection with segmental duodenectomy and preservation of the gastroduodenal artery. Hepatogastroenterology 1998; 45: 533–535.
132. Nakao A, Fernández-Cruz L. Pancreatic head resection with segmental duodenectomy: safety and long-term results. Ann Surg 2007; 246: 923–931.
133. Conci S, Ruzzenente A, Bertuzzo F, et al. Total Dorsal Pancreatectomy, an Alternative to Total Pancreatectomy: Report of a New Case and Literature Review. Digestive surgery. 2018 Jul 13: 1-6. doi: 10.1159/000490198. PubMed PMID: 30007967; eng.
134. Thayer SP, Fernandez-del Castillo C, Balcom JH, Warshaw AL: Complete dorsal pancreatectomy with preservation of the ventral pancreas: a new surgical technique. Surgery 2002; 131: 577–580.
135. Talbot ML, Foulis AK, Imrie CW: Total dorsal pancreatectomy for intraductal papillary mucinous neoplasm in a patient with pancreas divisum. Pancreatology 2005; 5(2–3): 285–288.
136. Scatton O, Sauvanet A, Cazals-Hatem D, Vullierme MP, Ruszniewski P, Belghiti J: Dorsal pancreatectomy: an embryology-based resection. J Gastrointest Surg 2006; 10: 434–438.
137. Bellin MD, Abu-El-Haija M, Morgan K, et al. A multicenter study of total pancreatectomy with islet autotransplantation (TPIAT): POST (Prospective Observational Study of TPIAT). Pancreatology: official journal of the International Association of Pancreatology (IAP) [et

al.]. 2018 Apr; 18(3): 286-290. doi: 10.1016/j.pan.2018.02.001. PubMed PMID: 29456124; PubMed Central PMCID: PMCPMC5879010; eng.
138. Bellin MD, Kerdsirichairat T, Beilman GJ, et al. Total Pancreatectomy With Islet Autotransplantation Improves Quality of Life in Patients With Refractory Recurrent Acute Pancreatitis. Clinical gastroenterology and hepatology: the official clinical practice journal of the American Gastroenterological Association. 2016 Sep; 14(9): 1317-23. doi: 10.1016/j.cgh.2016.02.027. PubMed PMID: 26965843; PubMed Central PMCID: PMCPMC5538725; eng.
139. Wilson GC, Sutton JM, Salehi M, et al. Surgical outcomes after total pancreatectomy and islet cell autotransplantation in pediatric patients. Surgery. 2013 Oct; 154(4): 777-83; discussion 783-4. doi: 10.1016/j.surg.2013.07.003. PubMed PMID: 24074415; eng.
140. Wilson GC, Sutton JM, Smith MT, et al. Completion pancreatectomy and islet cell autotransplantation as salvage therapy for patients failing previous operative interventions for chronic pancreatitis. Surgery. 2015 Oct; 158(4): 872-8; discussion 879-80. doi: 10.1016/j.surg.2015.04.045. PubMed PMID: 26173686; eng.
141. Theodorides T. Annular pancreas [in French]. J Chirurg (Paris) 1964; 87: 445-62.
142. Chevillotte G, Sahel J, Raillat A, et al. Annular pancreas. Report of one case associated with acute pancreatitis and diagnosed by endoscopic retrograde pancreatography. Dig Dis Sci 1984; 29: 75-7.
143. Glazer GM, Margulis AR. Annular pancreas: etiology and diagnosis using endoscopic retrograde cholangiopancreatography. Radiology 1979; 133: 303-6.
144. Tieken T. Annular pancreas. Am Med. 1901; 2: 826
145. Dowsett JF, Rode J, Russell RCG. Annular pancreas: a clinical, endoscopic, and immunohistochemical study. Gut. 1989; 30: 130–5.
146. Lloyd-Jones W, Mountain JC, Warren KW. Annular pancreas in the adult. Ann Surg. 1972; 176: 163–70.
147. Lecco TM. Zur morphologie des pancreas annulare. Sitzungsb Wien Akad Wiss Math-Nat KI. 1910; 119: 391–406.
148. Baldwin WM. A specimen of annular pancreas. Anat Rec. 1910; 4: 299–304.
149. Kamisawa T, Yuyang T, Egawa N, Ishiwata J, Okamoto A. A new embryologic hypothesis of annular pancreas. Hepatogastroenterology. 2001; 48: 277–8.
150. Fiocca R, Sessa F, Tenti P, et al. Pancreatic polypeptide (PP) cells in the PP-rich lobe of the human pancreas are identified ultrastructurally

and immunocytochemically as F cells. Histochemistry. 1983; 77: 511–23.

151. Suda K. Immunohistochemical and gross dissection studies of annular pancreas. Acta Pathol Jpn. 1990; 40: 505–8.
152. Yogi, Y., Shibue, T., Hashimoto, S., 1987. Annular pancreas detected in adults, diagnosed by endoscopic retrograde cholangiopancreatography: report of four cases. Gastroenterol. Jpn. 22, 92–99.
153. Fu, P.F., Yu, J.R., Liu, X.S., Shen, Q.Y., Zheng, S.S., 2005. Symptomatic adult annular pancreas: report of two cases and a review of the literature. Hepatobiliary Pancreat. Dis. Int. 4, 468–471.
154. Fukai M, Kamisawa T, Horiguchi SI, Hishima T, Kuruma S, Chiba K, Koizumi S,Tabata T, Nagao S, Kikuyama M, Honda G, Kurata M. A case of annular pancreas with Wirsung's duct encircling the duodenum: embryological hypothesis based on cholangiopancreatographic and immunohistochemical findings. Clin J Gastroenterol.2017 Jun; 10(3): 283-288. doi: 10.1007/s12328-017-0739-y. Epub 2017 Mar 31. PubMed PMID: 28364316.
155. Hebrok, M., Kim, S.K., St. Jacques, B., McMahon, A.P., Melton, D.A., 2000. Regulation of pancreas development by hedgehog signaling. Development 127, 4905–4913.
156. Ramalho-Santos, M., Melton, D.A., McMahon, A.P., 2000. Hedgehog signals regulate multiple aspects of gastrointestinal development. Development 127, 2763–2772.
157. Montgomery, R.C., Poindexter, M.H., Hall, G.H., Leigh, J.E., 1971. Report of a case of annular pancreas of the newborn in two consecutive siblings. Pediatrics 48, 148–149.
158. Jackson, L.G., Apostolides, P., 1978. Autosomal dominant inheritance of annular pancreas. Am. J. Med. Genet. 1, 319–321.
159. Hendricks, S.K., Sybert, V.P., 1991. Association of annular pancreas and duodenal obstruction—evidence for Mendelian inheritance? Clin. Genet. 39, 383–385.
160. Moon SB. "Ductal adenocarcinoma in annular pancreas": is it really an annular pancreas with pancreatic cancer? Int J Surg 2015; 24: 7e8
161. Benassai G, Perrotta S, Furino E, De Werra C, Aloia S, Del Giudice R, et al. Ductal adenocarcinoma in anular pancreas. International Journal of Surgery (2015), Int J Surg 2015; 21(Suppl 1): S95e7.
162. Foo FJ, Gill U, Verbeke CS, et al. Ampullary carcinoma associated with an annular pancreas. JOP 2007; 8: 50–54.
163. Nagpal SJS, Peeraphatdit T, Sannapaneni SK, Sharma A, Takahashi N, Kendrick ML, Majumder S, Vege SS. Clinical spectrum of adult

patients with annular pancreas: Findings from a large single institution cohort. Pancreatology. 2019 Mar; 19(2): 290-295. doi: 10.1016/j.pan.2018.12.009. Epub 2019 Jan 3. PubMed PMID: 30660391.
164. Drey, N.M., 1957. Symptomatic annular pancreas in the adult. Ann. Intern. Med. 46, 750–752.
165. Boomsma, J.H., Weemhoff, R.A., Polman, H.A., 1982. Sonographic appearance of annular pancreas in utero. A case report. Diagn. Imaging 51, 288–290.
166. Weiss, H., Sherer, D.M., Manning, F.A., 1999. Ultrasonography of fetal annular pancreas. Obstet. Gynecol. 94, 852.
167. Dankovcik, R., Muranska, S., Kucera, E., Jirasek, J.E., Feyereisl, J., Sudak, M., Dudas, M., 2010. Prenatal three-dimensional sonographic findings associated with annular pancreas. Fetal Diagn. Ther. 27, 57–60.
168. Dankovcik, R., Jirasek, J.E., Kucera, E., Feyereisl, J., Radonak, J., Dudas, M., 2008. Prenatal diagnosis of annular pancreas: reliability of the double bubble sign with periduodenal hyperechogenic band. Fetal Diagn. Ther. 24, 483–490.
169. Yang B, He F, He Q, Wang Z, Fang Q, Zhong W, Wang H. Diagnostic value of the acute angle between the prestenotic and poststenotic duodenum in neonatal annular pancreas. Eur Radiol. 2019 Jun; 29(6): 2902-2909. doi: 10.1007/s00330-018-5922-0. Epub 2019 Jan 7. PubMed PMID: 30617479.
170. Fantoni PA, Kaluso G, Sequenzia S, et al. Duodenal stenosis from intramural cystic annular pancreas. Hepatogastroenterology 1996; 43: 776–778.
171. Johnston DW. Annular pancreas: a new classification and clinical observations. Can J Surg 1978; 21: 241–244
172. Kalaitzakis E, Thorlacius H. Portal Annular Pancreas With Retroportal Pancreatic Duct Diagnosed With Endoscopic Ultrasound. Clin Gastroenterol Hepatol. 2015 Dec; 13(13): e175-6. doi: 10.1016/j.cgh.2015.04.026. Epub 2015 Apr 30. PubMed PMID: 25937363.
173. Joseph P, Raju RS, Vyas FL, et al. Portal annular pancreas. A rare variant and a new classification. JOP 2010; 11: 453–455.
174. Leyndecker JR, Baginski SG. Complete pancreatic encasement of the portal vein (circumportal pancreas): imaging findings and implications of a rare pancreatic anomaly. J Comput Assist Tomogr 2008; 32: 61–64.

175. Harnoss JM, Harnoss JC, DienerMK, et al. Portal annular pancreas. A systematic review of a clinical challenge. Pancreas 2014; 43: 981–986.
176. Kilbride H, Castor C, Andrews W. Congenital duodenal obstruction: timing of diagnosis during the newborn period. J Perinatol. 2010; 30: 197–200.
177. Gluer S, Petersen C, Ure BM. Simultaneous correction of duodenal atresia due to annular pancreas and malrotation by laparoscopy. Eur J Pediatr Surg. 2002; 12: 423–5.
178. Riquelme M, Aranda A, Riquelme-Q M, Rodriquez C. Laparoscopic treatment of duodenal obstruction: report on first experiences in Latin America. Eur J Pediatr Surg. 2008; 18: 334–6.
179. Jimenez JC, Emil S, Podnos Y, Nguyen N: Annular pancreas in children: a recent decade's experience. J Pediatr Surg; 39: 1654-1657.
180. Merrill JR, Raffensperger JG: Pediatric annular pancreas: twenty years' experience. J Pediatr Surg; 11: 921-925.
181. Li B, Chen WB, Wang SQ, Wang YB. Laparoscopic diagnosis and treatment of neonates with duodenal obstruction associated with an annular pancreas: report of 11 cases. Surg Today. 2015 Jan; 45(1): 17-21. doi: 10.1007/s00595-014-0850-3. Epub 2014 Jan 30. PubMed PMID: 24477526.
182. Hyden WH. The true nature of annular pancreas. Ann Surg 1963; 157: 71e7.
183. Thomford NR, Knight PR, Pace WG, Madura JA. Annular pancreas in the adult: selection of operation. Ann Surg 1972; 176: 159e62.
184. Ulusan S, Bal N, Kizilkilic O, Bolat F, Yildirim S, Yildirim T et al. Case report: solid-pseudopapillary tumor of the pancreas associated with dorsal agenesis. Br J Radiol 2005; 78: 441–3.
185. Macari M, Giovanniello G, Blair L, Krinsky G. Diagnosis of agenesis of the dorsal pancreas with MR pancreatography. AJR Am J Roentgenol 1998; 170: 144–6.
186. Schnedl WJ, Piswanger-Soelkner C, Wallner SJ, Reittner P, Krause R, Lipp RW, et al. Agenesis of the dorsal pancreas and associated diseases. Dig Dis Sci 2009; 54: 481–487.
187. Heiberg KA. Ein Fall von fehlender Cauda pancreatis (bei einem Diabetiker). Centralbl Allg Pathol Patholog Anat 1911; 22: 676-7.
188. A Cienfuegos J, Rotellar F, Salguero J, Benito A, Solórzano JL, Sangro B. Agenesis of the dorsal pancreas: systematic review of a clinical challenge. Rev Esp Enferm Dig. 2016 Aug; 108(8): 479-84. doi: 10.17235/reed.2016.4474/2016. Review. PubMed PMID: 27468966.

189. Schnedl WJ, Reisinger EC, Schreiber F, et al. Complete and partial agenesis of the dorsal pancreas within one family. Gastrointest Endosc 1995; 42(5): 485-7. DOI: 10.1016/S0016-5107(95)70055-2
190. Haldorsen IS, Raeder H, Vesterhus M, et al. The role of pancreatic imaging in monogenic diabetes mellitus. Nat Rev Endocrinol 2011; 8(3): 148-59. DOI: 10.1038/nrendo.2011.197
191. Body-Bechou D, Loget P, D'Herve D, et al. TCF2/HNF-1beta mutations: 3 cases of fetal severe pancreatic agenesis or hypoplasia and multicystic renal dysplasia. Prenat Diagn 2014; 34(1): 90-3. DOI: 10.1002/pd.4264.
192. Rittenhouse DW, Kennedy EP, Mascaro AA, et al. The novel triad of dorsal agenesis of the pancreas with concurrent pancreatic ductal adenocarcinoma and nonalcoholic chronic calcific pancreatitis: A case series and review of the literature. J Gastrointest Surg 2011; 15(9): 1643-9. DOI: 10.1007/s11605-011-1542-6.
193. Lang K, Lasson A, Muller MF, et al. Dorsal agenesis of the pancreas - A rare cause of abdominal pain and insulin-dependent diabetes. Acta Radiol 2012; 53(1): 2-4. DOI: 10.1258/ar.2011.110480.
194. Dor Y, Brown J, Martínez OI, et al. Adult pancreatic beta-cells are formed by self-duplication rather than stem-cell differentiation. Nature 2004; 429(6987): 41-6. DOI: 10.1038/nature02520.
195. Ionescu-Tirgoviste C, Gagniuc PA, Gubceac E, et al. A 3D map of the islet routes throughout the healthy human pancreas. Sci Rep 2015; 5: 14634. DOI: 10.1038/srep14634.
196. Sakpal SV, Sexcius L, Babel N, et al. Agenesis of the dorsal pancreas and its association with pancreatic tumors. Pancreas 2009; 38(4): 367-73. DOI: 10.1097/MPA.0b013e318196c401.
197. Sannappa RM, Buragohain J, Sarma D, et al. Agenesis of dorsal pancreas associated with periampullary pancreaticobiliary type adenocarcinoma. JOP 2014; 15(5): 489-92.
198. Murtaugh LC, Keefe MD. Regeneration and repair of the exocrine pancreas. Annu Rev Physiol 2015; 77: 229-49. DOI: 10.1146/annurevphysiol-021014-071727.
199. Riguetto CM, Pelichek S, Moura Neto A. Heterotaxy syndrome with agenesis of dorsal pancreas and diabetes mellitus: case report and review of the literature. Arch Endocrinol Metab. 2019 May 30; 63(4): 445-448. doi: 10.20945/2359-3997000000142. PMID: 31166366.
200. Suh PS, Lee JH, Yu JS, Hee Kim J, Kim B, Kim HJ, Huh J, Kim JK, Lee D. Three cases of pancreatic pseudocysts associated with dorsal pancreatic agenesis. Radiol Case Rep. 2018 Oct 23; 14(1): 79-82.

doi: 10.1016/j.radcr.2018.09.023.eCollection 2019 Jan. PubMed PMID: 30377453; PubMed Central PMCID: PMC6202790.

201. Lal H, Yadav P, Mourya C. Dependent stomach sign and dependent intestine sign of dorsal pancreatic agenesis. Abdom Radiol (NY). 2017 Feb; 42(2): 667-669. doi: 10.1007/s00261-016-0911-8. Review. PubMed PMID: 27654989.
202. Soyer P, Spelle L, Pelage J, Dufresne A, Rondeau Y, Gouhiri M, et al. (1999) Cystic fibrosis in adolescents and adults: fatty replacement of the pancreas—CT evaluation and functional correlation. Radiology 210(3): 611–615. doi: 10.1148/radiology.210.3.r99mr08611.
203. Yamauchi FI, Ortega CD, Blasbalg R, Rocha MS, Jukemura J, Cerri GG (2012) Multidetector CT evaluation of the postoperative pancreas. RadioGraphics 32(3): 743–764. doi: 10.1148/rg.323105121.
204. Dinkhauser P, Paesold J, Hubner D, Steffan V, Lampl R, Hofer H. Agenesis of the dorsal pancreas: a very rare entity causing diabetes mellitus. Wien Med Wochenschr. 2020 May; 170(7-8): 168-170. doi: 10.1007/s10354-019-00717-1. Epub 2019 Dec 3. PMID: 31797244.
205. Kawasaki S, Itoi T, Iwasaki E, Hosoe N, Ogata H, Kanai T. Successful Pancreatic Duct Stent Placement for Recurrent Pancreatitis in a Patient with Polysplenia with Agenesis of the Dorsal Pancreas and Peutz-Jeghers Syndrome. Intern Med. 2016; 55(13): 1743-6. doi: 10.2169/internalmedicine.55.6128. Epub 2016 Jul 1. PMID: 27374675.
206. Dumitraşcu T, Scarlat A, Diaconescu A, Ionescu M. Dorsal pancreas agenesis and ductal adenocarcinoma: surgical implications of an extremely rare association. Chirurgia (Bucur). 2012 May-Jun; 107(3): 389-92. PMID: 22844839.
207. Mortele K.J., Rocha T.C., Streeter J.L., Taylor A.J. (2006) Multimodality imaging of pancreatic and biliary congenital anomalies. Radiographics 26: 715-731.
208. Sotirios, K., Dimitrios, F., & Panagiotis, S. (2019). Ansa pancreatica. Review of the literature. Italian Journal of Anatomy and Embryology, 124(1), 79-86.
209. Jarrar M.S., Khenissi A., Ghrissi R., Hamila F., Letaief R. (2013) Ansa pancreatica: an anatomic variation and a rare cause of acute pancreatitis. Surg. Radiol. Anat. 35: 745-748.
210. Houssem Harbi MD, Nozha Toumi MD, Mohamed Ben Amar MD, Acute Pancreatitis due to a rare ductal anomaly: ansa pancreatica, The American Journal of the Medical Sciences (2018).
211. Bajaji A. Bisection, Disjuncture, Aqueduct: Pancreas Divisum. Gastroenterol Hepatol Int J 2018, 3(1): 000138.

212. Dawson W, Langman J. An anatomical-radiological study on the pancreatic duct pattern in man. Anat Rec. 1961; 139: 59–68.
213. Kamisawa T., Yuyang T., Egawa N., Ishiwata J., Okamoto A. (1998) Patency of the accessory pancreatic duct in relation to its course and shape: a dye-injection endoscopic retrograde pancreatography study. Am. J. Gastroenterol. 93: 2135-2140.
214. Liessi F., Manfredi R., Liessi G., Pozzi-Mucelli R (2010) Anatomical variants of the pancreatic ducts. Proc. European Congress of Radiology: C-0174 (12 pages); doi: 10.1594/ecr2010/C-0174.
215. Adibelli Z.H., Adatepe M., Imamoglu C., Esen O.S., Erkan N., Yildirim M. (2016) Anatomic variations of the pancreatic duct and their relevance with the Cambridge classification system: MRCP findings of 1158 consecutive patients. Radiol. Oncol. 50: 370-377.
216. Hayashi T.Y., Gonoi W., Yoshikawa T., Hayashi N., Ohtomo K. (2016) Ansa pancreatica as a predisposing factor for recurrent acute pancreatitis. World.J. Gastroenterol.22: 89408948.
217. Narayanan G., Shabna C. (2017) Variations in the duct system of the pancreas: a cadaveric study. Int. J. Anat. Res. 5: 4136-4143.
218. Fatima Hussain SN, Malik MI, Khan SA. Case report on Ansa Pancreatica: An Uncommon Cause Accounting for Recurrent Pancreatitis in Children. J Pak Med Assoc. 2019; 69(11): 1759-1761. doi: 10.5455/JPMA.29846.
219. Kim HM, Park JY, Kim MJ. Ansa Pancreatica: A Case Report of a Type of Ductal Variation in a Patient with Idiopathic Acute Recurrent Pancreatitis. J Korean Soc Radiol 2010; 63: 83-6.
220. Bhasin D.K., Rana S.S., Nanda M., Gupta R., Nagi B., Wig J.D. (2006) Ansa pancreatica type of ductal anatomy in a patient with idiopathic acute pancreatitis. J. Pancreas (JOP) 7: 315-320.
221. Jagielski M., Smoczyński M., Drelich-Góreczna B., Adrych K. (2017) Transduodenal drainage of symptomatic walled-off pancreatic necrosis in a patient with ansa pancreatica anatomic variation. Arch. Med. Sci. 13: 267-269.
222. Ishii H., Arai K., Fukushima M., Maruoka Y., Hoshino M., Nakamura A., Koike Y., Sakamoto N., Hanada H., Kusano M., Okamatsu, T. (1998) Fusion variations of pancreatic ducts in patients with anomalous arrangement of pancreaticobiliary ductal system. J. Hepatobiliary Pancreat. Surg. 5: 327-332.
223. Tanaka T., Ichiba Y., Miura Y., Itoh H., Dohi K. (1991) Variations of the pancreatic ducts as a cause of chronic alcoholic pancreatitis. Am. J. Gastroenterol. 86: 792-793.

224. Tanaka T., Ichiba Y., Miura Y., Itoh H., Dohi K. (1992) Variations of the pancreatic ducts as a cause of chronic alcoholic pancreatitis; ansa pancreatica. Am. J. Gastroenterol. 87: 806.
225. Bülow R., Simon P., Thiel R., Thamm P., Messner P., Lerch M.M., Mayerle J., Völzke H., Hosten N., Kühn J.P. (2014) Anatomic variants of the pancreatic duct and their clinical relevance: an MR-guided study in the general population. Eur. Radiol. 24: 3142-3149.
226. Tamura R., Ishibashi T., Takahashi S. (2006) Chronic pancreatitis: MRCP versus ERCP for quantitative caliber measurement and qualitative evaluation. Radiology 238: 920-928.
227. Hichem Ayari et al. L'ansa pancreatica: une cause rare de pancréatite aigue. Pan African Medical Journal. 2012; 13: 33. [doi: 10.11604/pamj.2012.13.33.1462]
228. López-Durán S, Zaera C, González-Martín JA, Foruny JR, Albillos A, Vázquez-Sequeiros E. The endoscopic ultrasound-assisted Rendez-Vous technique for treatment of recurrent pancreatitis due to pancreas divisum and ansa pancreatica. Rev Esp Enferm Dig 2017; 109(11): 798-800. DOI: 10.17235/reed.2017.4949/2017.